PLAB 2 : 100 OBJECTIVE STRUCTURED CLINICAL EXAMINATIONS

I dedicate this book to my husband, William,
and to my three daughters, Olivia, Emily and Henrietta

PLAB 2: 100 OBJECTIVE STRUCTURED CLINICAL EXAMINATIONS

By

Una F. Coales
BA MD FRCS (ED) FRCS (OTO) DRCOG
Senior House Officer
Department of Obstetrics and Gynaecology
King's College Hospital
Denmark Hill
London, UK

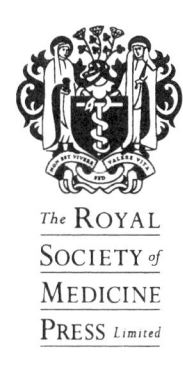

The ROYAL
SOCIETY of
MEDICINE
PRESS Limited

© 2001 Royal Society of Medicine Press Ltd
Reprinted 2003, 2004

1 Wimpole Street, London W1G 0AE
207 Westminster Road, Lake Forest, IL 60045, USA
www.rsmpress.co.uk

Apart from any fair dealing for the purposes of research or private study, or criticism or review, as permitted under the UK Copyright, Designs and Patents Act 1988, no part of this publication may be reprinted, stored, or transmitted, in any form or by any means, without the prior permission in writing of the publishers or in the case of reprographic reproduction in accordance with the terms or licences issued by the appropriate Reproduction Organisation outside the UK. Enquiries concerning reproduction outside the terms stated here should be sent to the publishers at the UK address printed on this page.

The right of Una Coales to be identified as author of this work has been asserted by her in accordance with the Copyright, Designs and Patents Act 1988.

British Library Cataloguing in Publication Data
A catalogue record for this book is available from the British Library

ISBN: 1-85315-503-9

Typeset by Phoenix Photosetting, Chatham, Kent

Printed in Great Britain by Bell and Bain Ltd, Glasgow

Contents

Preface	vii
Acknowledgements	ix
Recommended texts and references	xi
Stations	1
Answers	101

Preface

I was trained in the USA (The Johns Hopkins University and The Oregon Health Sciences University School of Medicine) and relocated to the UK to practice surgery. Like you, the reader, I was offered no recommended textbooks or courses and was required to sit and subsequently passed the Professional and Linguistic Assessments Boards (PLAB) test under its old guise. As of July 2000, this format was preceded by PLAB Parts 1 and 2. The present book is an adjunct to my definitive book on PLAB Part 1: *PLAB: 1000 Extended Matching Questions* (2000). It is the only book to date written on PLAB Part 2 and is offered in the identical format of the PLAB Part 2 Objective Structured Clinical Examination given by the General Medical Council (GMC). This book presents 100 objective structured clinical examinations (OSCEs) and covers the main skills tested in the OSCE examination – communication, history taking, clinical examination, practical skills and emergency management – as defined by the GMC.

To enter Part 2 (OSCE), the candidate must have successfully completed Part 1 of the PLAB examination, which consists of 200 extended matching questions. Part 2 consists of a 14-station OSCE and tests your clinical and communication skills over 1 hour 36 minutes, with 5 minutes allocated for each station. Each station consists of a number of objectives and will be graded A, excellent; B, good; C, adequate; D, fail; and E, severe fail. To pass Part 2, a candidate must obtain a minimum of grade C for ten stations and must not have received a grade E for more than one station. Part 2 must be taken within 2 years of having passed Part 1, and Part 2 (OSCE) is offered ten times a year in the UK. The candidate is offered four attempts to pass Part 2 and faces repeating the IELTS test and the entire PLAB test if he or she fails on the fourth attempt. As of April 2001, the cost of the Part 2 PLAB exam rose substantially from £150 to £430!

Take a deep breath! The PLAB test is not impossible to pass! Allow me to show you how. I strongly advise you to use this book in conjunction with a clinical attachment in Accident and Emergency in a district general hospital to practice and hone your clinical skills, and by doing so you will pass Part 2 of the PLAB test! Instead of paying exorbitant fees to a suspect PLAB 2 course, write to the clinical director or consultant in charge of an Accident and Emergency Department and ask permission to sit in for a month or two in the Accident and Emergency Department. The clinical director or consultant in charge will be flattered and honoured by your request, and you, in turn, will be of invaluable service to the busy senior house officers on duty. You will gain confidence to perform for the OSCEs in a fluent and professional manner. Having subsequently sat and passed the FRCS exams Part 1 and 2 in both General Surgery and Otolaryngology and the DRCOG exam, I have also come to realize that foreign medical postgraduates need to familiarize themselves with the British system of clinical examination and methods to reach a diagnosis. This is an added feature in this book and will facilitate passing future postgraduate examinations in the UK.

Una F. Coales
May 2001

Acknowledgements

I would like to thank the following doctors for their invaluable contribution to the content of *PLAB 2: 100 Objective Structured Clinical Examinations*:

Dr P. Gishen FRCR (Clinical Director and Consultant Radiologist at Hammersmith and Charing Cross Hospitals) for the use of several chest X-rays borrowed from the X-ray Museum Department, which he established at King's College Hospital.

Dr Hammad Malik MRCOphth for his input in the ophthalmology OSCEs.

Dr Stam Kapetanakis MRCP (Specialist Registrar in Cardiology at King's College Hospital) for his expert advice on electrocardiogram interpretation and the management of acute myocardial infarction.

Dr Rehan Salim MBBS (Research Fellow in Obstetrics and Gynaecology at King's College Hospital) and his wife, Dr Sheema Salim, who recently sat and passed PLAB Parts I and II.

Recommended texts and references

Surgery

Apley A.G. *et al.* (1993) *Apley's System of Orthopaedics and Fractures*, 7th edn. Arnold, London.

Browse N.L. (1991) *An Introduction to the Symptoms and Signs of Surgical Disease*, 2nd edn. Arnold, London.

Lattimer C.R. *et al.* (1996) *Key Topics in General Surgery*. BIOS, Oxford.

McLatchie G.R. (1990) *Oxford Handbook of Clinical Surgery*. Oxford University Press, Oxford.

Unwin A. *et al.* (1995) *Emergency Orthopaedics and Trauma*. Butterworth-Heinemann, Oxford.

Medicine

Fauci A. *et al.* (1997) *Harrison's Principles of Internal Medicine*, 14th edn. McGraw-Hill, New York.

Hope R.A. *et al.* (1998) *Oxford Handbook of Clinical Medicine*, 4th edn. Oxford University Press, Oxford.

Kumar P.J. *et al.* (1998) *Clinical Medicine*, 4th edn. Ballière Tindall, London.

Rubenstein D. *et al.* (1991) *Lecture Notes on Clinical Medicine*, 5th edn. Blackwell, Oxford.

Obstetrics and Gynaecology

Chamberlain G. & Hamilton-Fairly D. (1999) *Lecture Notes on Obstetrics and Gynaecology*. Blackwell, Oxford.

Hacker N.F. *et al.* (1998) *Essentials of Obstetrics and Gynaecology*, 3rd edn. W.B. Saunders, Philadelphia.

Rymer, J. *et al.* (1998) *Preparation and Revision for the DRCOG*, 2nd edn. Churchill Livingstone, London.

Psychiatry

Collier J.A.B. *et al.* (1991) *Oxford Handbook of Clinical Specialties*, 3rd edn. Oxford University Press, Oxford.

Otolaryngology

Roland N.J. *et al.* (1995) *Key Topics in Otolaryngology*. BIOS, Oxford.

Resuscitation

Jaffe A.S. *et al.* (1987) *Advanced Cardiac Life Support*, 2nd edn. American Heart Association, New York.

Alexander, R.H. & Proctor H.J. (1993) *Advanced Trauma Life Support*, 5th edn. American College of Surgeons, Chicago.

Station 1
Theme: Toe joint pain

This station tests your ability to take a history and reach a diagnosis.

Mr Johnson has been referred to you in the Rheumatology Clinic because he continues to have pain in his left great toe.

Take a relevant history and suggest a likely diagnosis.

This station lasts 5 minutes.

Station 2
Theme: Emergency contraception

This station tests your ability to take a history and suggest management.

Miss Miller is 15 years old and presents to Accident and Emergency requesting emergency contraception because she had unprotected sex 48 hours ago.

Take a relevant history and suggest appropriate management.

This station lasts 5 minutes.

Station 3
Theme: Interpreting an electrocardiogram

This station tests your ability to interpret accurately a 12-lead electrocardiogram.

A 40-year-old man presents to Casualty with acute onset of chest pain.

Interpret his 12-lead electrocardiogram. Is there cause to be concerned?

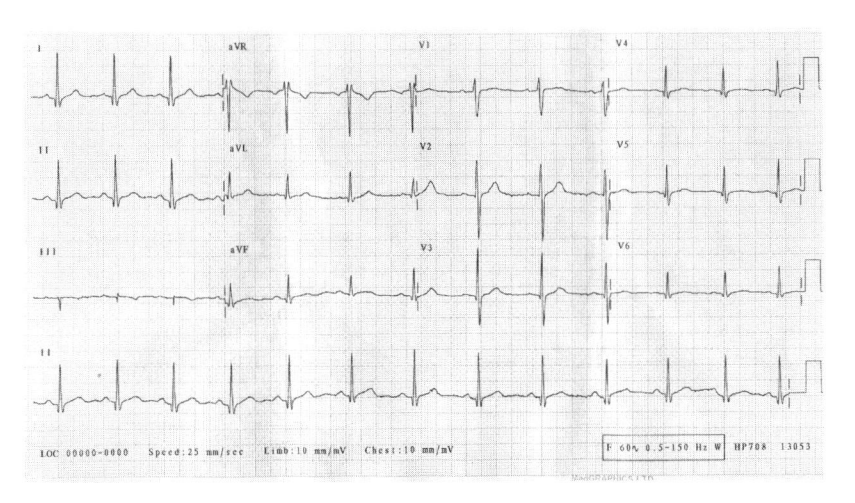

This station lasts 5 minutes.

Station 4
Theme: PV bleed

This station tests your ability to take a history and reach a diagnosis.

Mrs McGuire presents to Accident and Emergency with profuse bleeding per vagina.

Take a relevant history and suggest a likely diagnosis.

This station lasts 5 minutes.

Station 5
Theme: Ear pain

This station tests your ability to take a history and reach a diagnosis.

Miss White has been referred to you in the ENT Clinic with right-sided ear pain.

Take a relevant history and suggest a likely diagnosis to the examiner.

This station lasts 5 minutes.

Station 6
Theme: Interpretation of a chest X-ray

This station tests your ability to interpret a chest X-ray.

Mrs Markham is a 50-year-old woman who complains of shortness of breath and left-sided chest pain.

Interpret her chest X-ray.

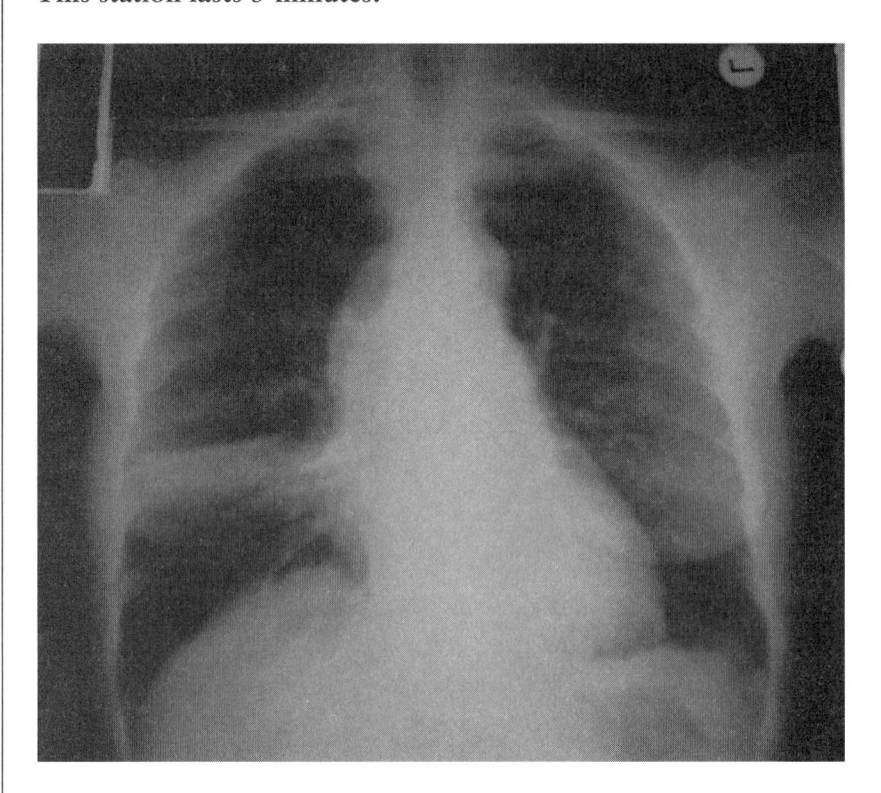

This station lasts 5 minutes.

Station 7
Theme: Examination of the ear

This station tests your ability to conduct a physical examination of the ear.

Mr Johnson presents with sudden onset of diminished hearing in the right ear.

Examine the ear.

This station lasts 5 minutes.

Station 8
Theme: Bladder catheterization

This station tests your ability to perform bladder catheterization.

Mr Thomas is a 65-year-old man who presents to Accident and Emergency unable to void for the past 24 hours. On examination, he has a tense bladder palpable at the level of the umbilicus. He is in urinary retention. You decide to catheterize his bladder.

Demonstrate bladder catheterization on the manikin.

This station lasts 5 minutes.

Equipment provided: male manikin, catheter trolley containing antiseptic cleansing fluid, sterile drapes, Foley size 12 urethral catheter, lignocaine gel, forceps, cotton balls, catheter bag and tubing, sterile gloves, 10 ml syringe with 10 ml ampoule of normal saline.

Station 9
Theme: Tubal sterilization

This station tests your ability to obtain informed consent.

Miss Jones is a 22-year-old woman with two children and would like to be sterilized. She has a history of autoimmune hepatitis and has had a liver transplant.

Obtain informed consent for tubal sterilization.

This station lasts 5 minutes.

Station 10
Theme: Interpreting an electrocardiogram

This station tests your ability to interpret accurately a 12-lead electrocardiogram.

A 62-year-old man is brought by ambulance to Casualty with severe chest pain. His blood pressure is 170/100. You are the Accident and Emergency SHO on duty.

Interpret his 12-lead electrocardiogram. Is there cause for concern?

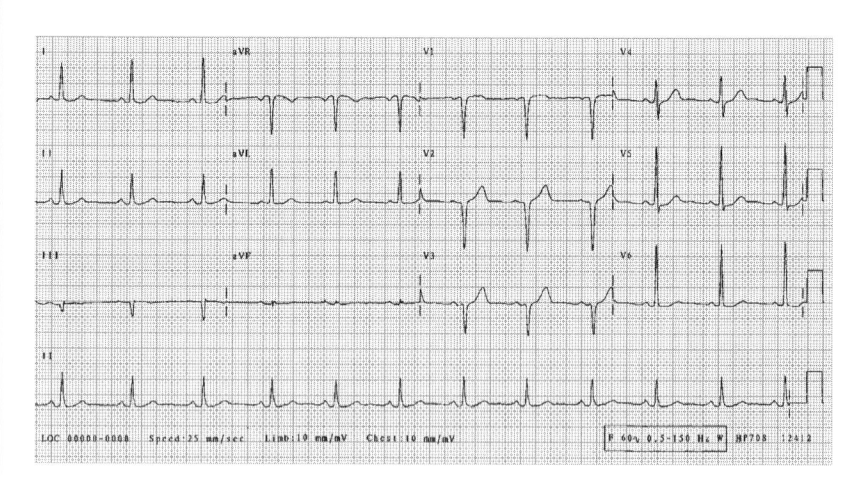

This station lasts 5 minutes.

Station 11
Theme: Basic life support

This station tests your skills in basic adult cardiopulmonary resuscitation.

You witness a 60-year-old man collapse in the middle of Hyde Park, London.

Perform basic adult cardiopulmonary resuscitation on the manikin.

This station lasts 5 minutes.

Station 12
Theme: Interpretation of a chest X-ray

This station tests your ability to interpret a chest X-ray.

Mr Henry is a 24-year-old airline steward who complains of fever and persistent dry cough.

Interpret his chest X-ray.

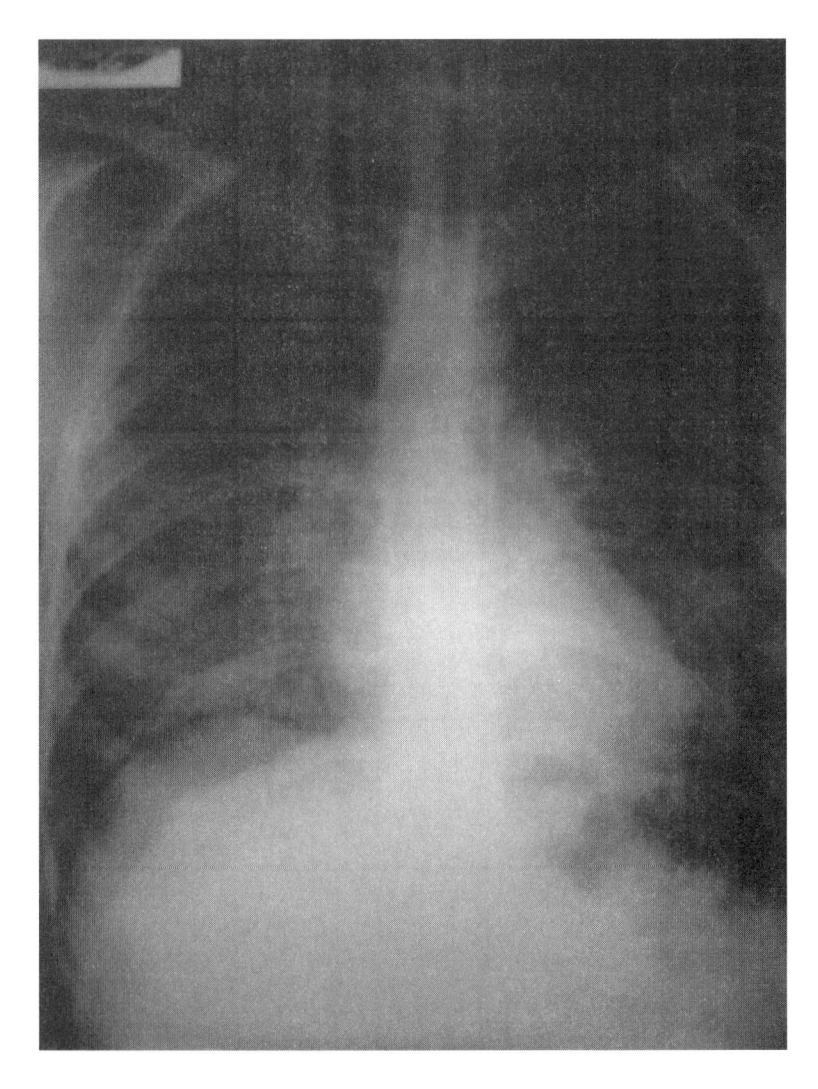

This station lasts 5 minutes.

Station 13
Theme: Knee examination

This station tests your ability to perform an examination of the knee.

A 20-year-old rugby player presents to Accident and Emergency complaining of a painful swollen right knee after twisting his leg at practice. He heard it 'pop' and could not continue weight bearing.

Examine the knee and suggest a likely diagnosis.

This station lasts 5 minutes.

Station 14
Theme: Taking a cervical smear

This station tests your ability to perform a speculum examination and obtain a cervical smear.

A 28-year-old woman presents in the Gynaecology Clinic and has not had a cervical smear in the past 3 years.

Perform a speculum examination and take a cervical smear on the manikin.

This station lasts 5 minutes.

Station 15
Theme: Venepuncture

This station tests your ability to perform venepuncture.

Miss Johnson attends your pre-assessment clinic and requires pre-operative blood tests. She is 38 years old, Nigerian and healthy. She is scheduled for myomectomy in 10 days.

Inform the patient which blood tests you will be taking and perform venepuncture on the manikin.

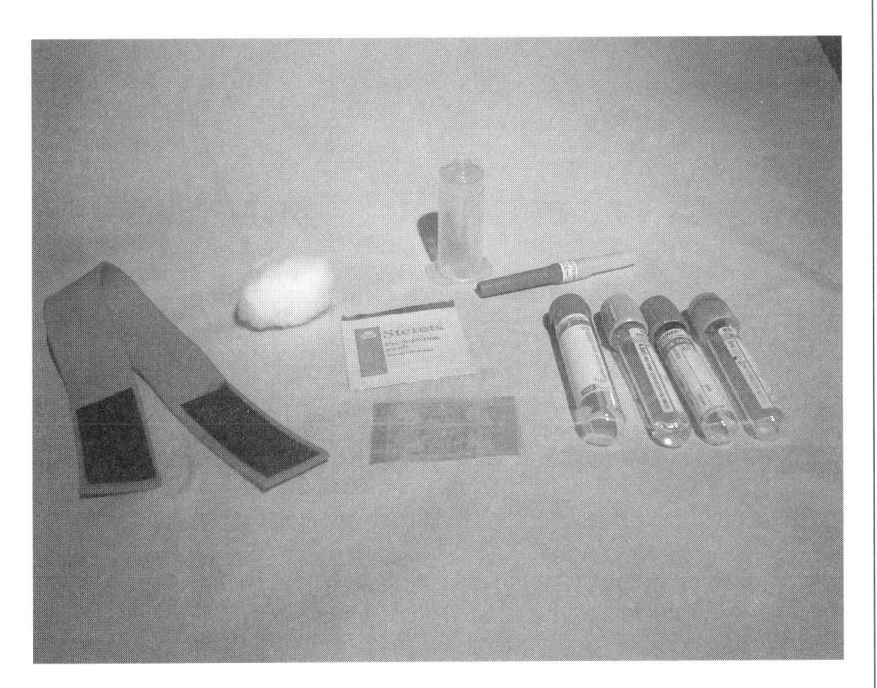

This station lasts 5 minutes.

Station 16
Theme: Interpreting an electrocardiogram

This station tests your ability to interpret accurately a 12-lead electrocardiogram.

A 62-year-old man presents to Casualty with chest pains. He also describes his heart as pounding in his chest.

Interpret his 12-lead electrocardiogram. Mention the rate, rhythm and describe the abnormalities.

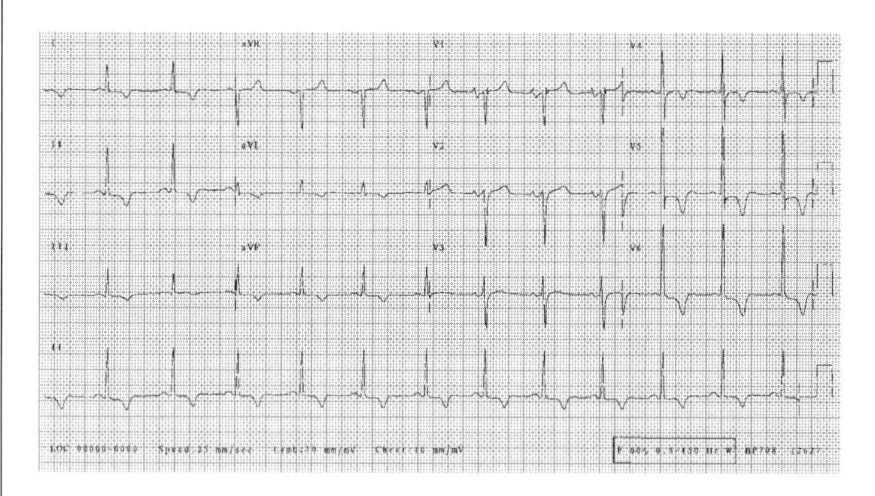

This station lasts 5 minutes.

Station 17
Theme: Suturing

This station tests your skills in suturing and your knowledge of suture material.

A 62-year-old woman has cut her leg 2 hours ago while gardening. She requires sutures to the open wound. Her tetanus immunization is up to date.

Using the plastic model of a leg, demonstrate the technique of suturing.

This station lasts 5 minutes.

Station 18
Theme: Giving advice on hormone replacement therapy

This station tests your ability to offer advice on hormone replacement therapy (HRT).

Mrs Markham is a 50-year-old woman who has been referred to you in Gynaecology Clinic because she suffers from hot flushes, night sweats, urinary frequency and mood swings. She has been amenorrhoeic for a year.

Discuss the benefits and risks of HRT.

This station lasts 5 minutes.

Station 19
Theme: Interpretation of a chest X-ray

This station tests your ability to interpret a chest X-ray.

Mr Oborne is a 40-year-old man who complains of a persistent cough.

Interpret his chest X-ray.

This station lasts 5 minutes.

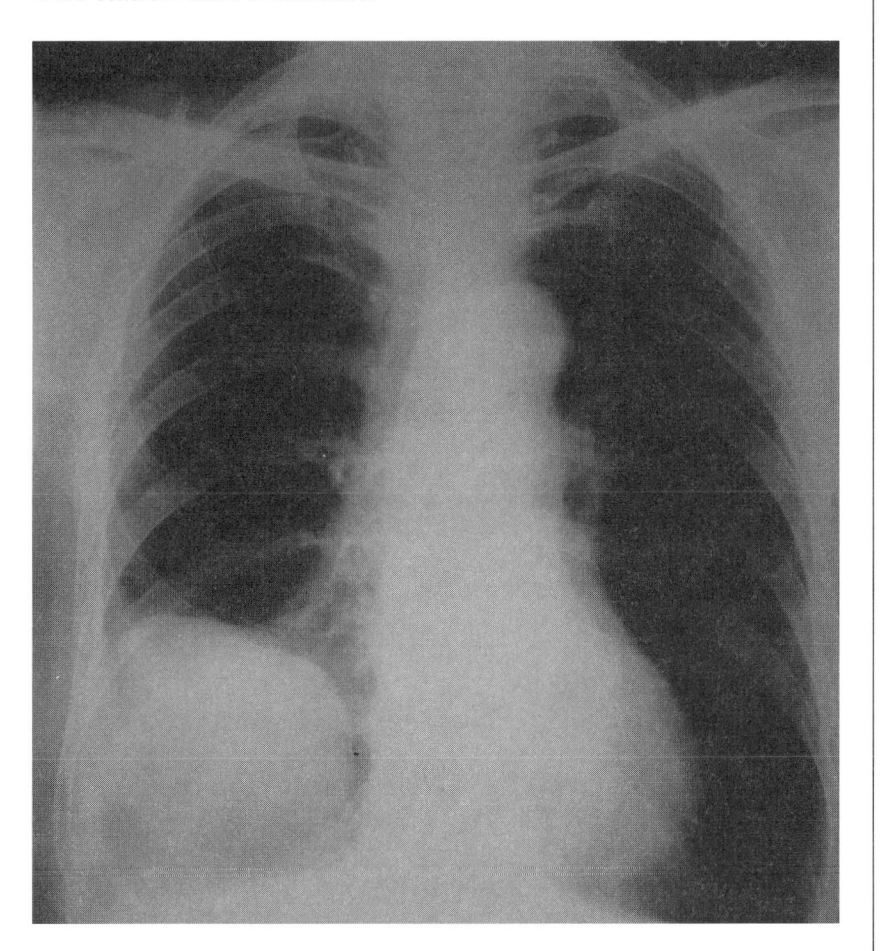

Station 20
Theme: Interpreting an electrocardiogram

This station tests your ability to interpret accurately a 12-lead electrocardiogram.

A 65-year-old woman presents to Casualty with chest pain.

Interpret her 12-lead electrocardiogram. Is there cause for concern?

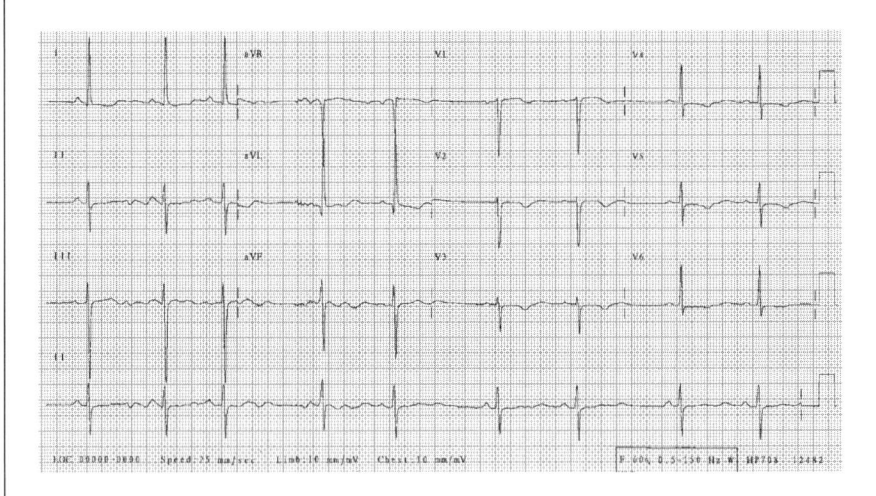

This station lasts 5 minutes.

Station 21
Theme: Emergency management of diabetic ketoacidosis

This station tests your ability to manage diabetic ketoacidosis.

A 60-year-old diabetic man is brought by ambulance to Casualty. He is drowsy. His blood pressure is 90/60. His respiratory rate is 30 breaths per minute. He has dry mucous membranes and acetone breath. His wife informs you that he has not been taking his insulin regularly.

Manage the patient appropriately.

This station lasts 5 minutes.

Station 22
Theme: Interpreting an electrocardiogram

This station tests your ability to interpret accurately a 12-lead electrocardiogram.

A 72-year-old woman presents to Casualty complaining of chest pain.

Interpret her 12-lead electrocardiogram. Is there cause for concern?

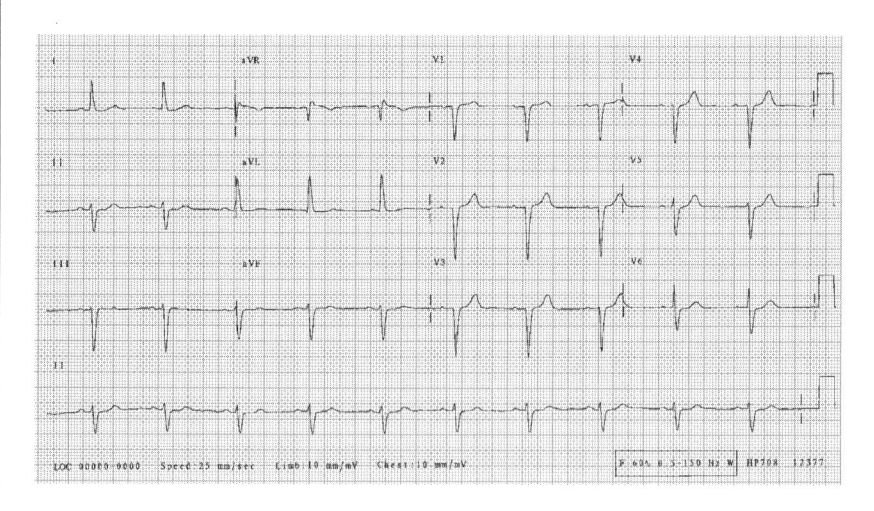

This station lasts 5 minutes.

Station 23
Theme: Mental State Examination

This station tests your ability to perform a Mental State Examination.

Mr Rowe is a 75-year-old man who is brought to Accident and Emergency by his daughter who reports that he is not himself.

Perform a Mental State Examination and document your findings. You will also be marked for your ability to maintain effective records.

This station lasts 5 minutes.

Station 24
Theme: Examination of the abdomen

This station tests your ability to perform a competent examination of the abdomen.

Mr Jones is a 55-year-old alcoholic who presents with right-sided upper abdominal discomfort.

Perform an examination of his abdomen and examine for signs of chronic liver disease.

This station lasts 5 minutes.

Station 25
Theme: Interpreting an electrocardiogram

This station tests your ability to interpret accurately a 12-lead electrocardiogram.

A 60-year-old man is being seen in pre-assessment clinic for a hernia operation. You send him off for a 12-lead electrocardiogram. He returns with his electrocardiogram in hand.

Interpret his 12-lead electrocardiogram. Mention the rate, rhythm and any abnormalities.

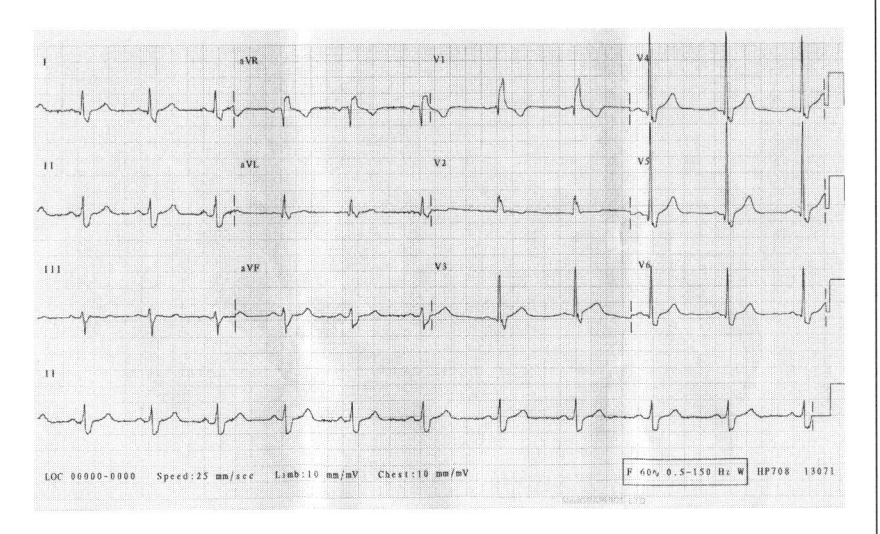

This station lasts 5 minutes.

Station 26
Theme: Examination of the eye

This station tests your ability to perform a satisfactory eye examination.

Mrs Jones is a 72-year-old woman who wears glasses for long-sightedness. She complains that since 8 p.m., she has been vomiting and her vision is worse. She also has red eyes.

Perform an eye examination and make a reasonable diagnosis.

This station lasts 5 minutes.

Station 27
Theme: Interpretation of a chest X-ray

This station tests your ability to interpret a chest X-ray.

Mrs Brock is a 65-year-old woman post-nephrectomy who is having difficulty breathing. She had just been advanced to a soft diet.

Interpret her chest X-ray.

This station lasts 5 minutes.

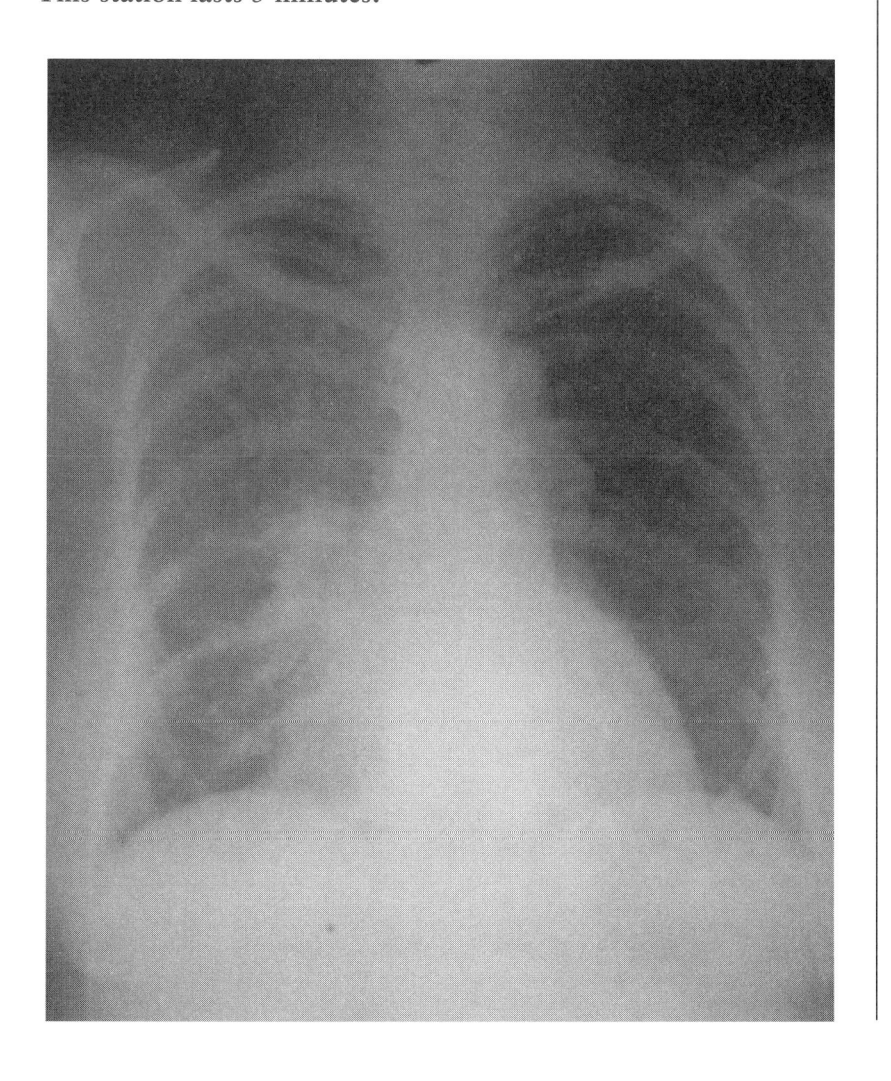

Station 28
Theme: Interpreting an electrocardiogram

This station tests your ability to interpret accurately a 12-lead electrocardiogram.

A 70-year-old man presents to Casualty with severe epistaxis. He is on warfarin. You are the ENT SHO. His epistaxis is not controlled with packing. INR is 2.0. Your registrar has decided to take him to theatre. You arrange an urgent preoperative 12-lead electrocardiogram. What has the patient omitted to inform you? Should you stop his warfarin?

Interpret his 12-lead electrocardiogram.

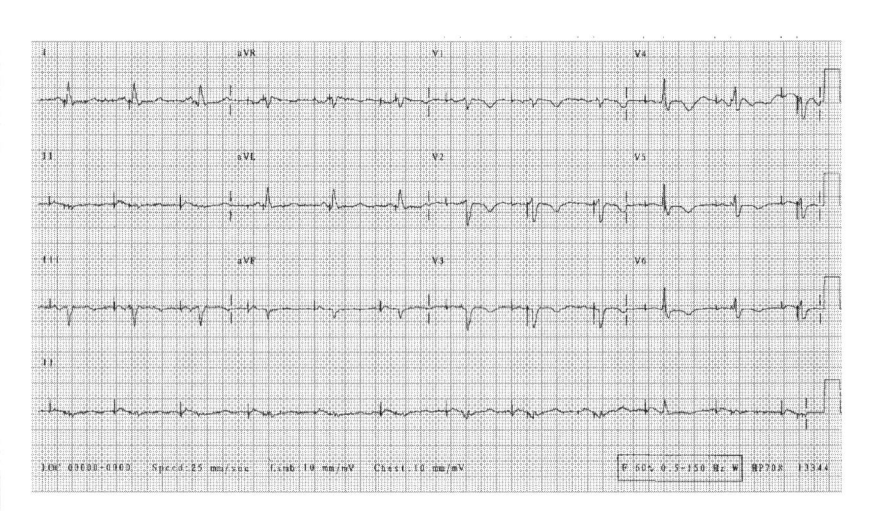

This station lasts 5 minutes.

Station 29
Theme: Taking a blood pressure

This station tests your ability to take an accurate blood pressure.

Mr Smythson is a 60-year-old man who complains of feeling faint. He states he nearly passed out when he was on the toilet this morning.

Take his blood pressure.

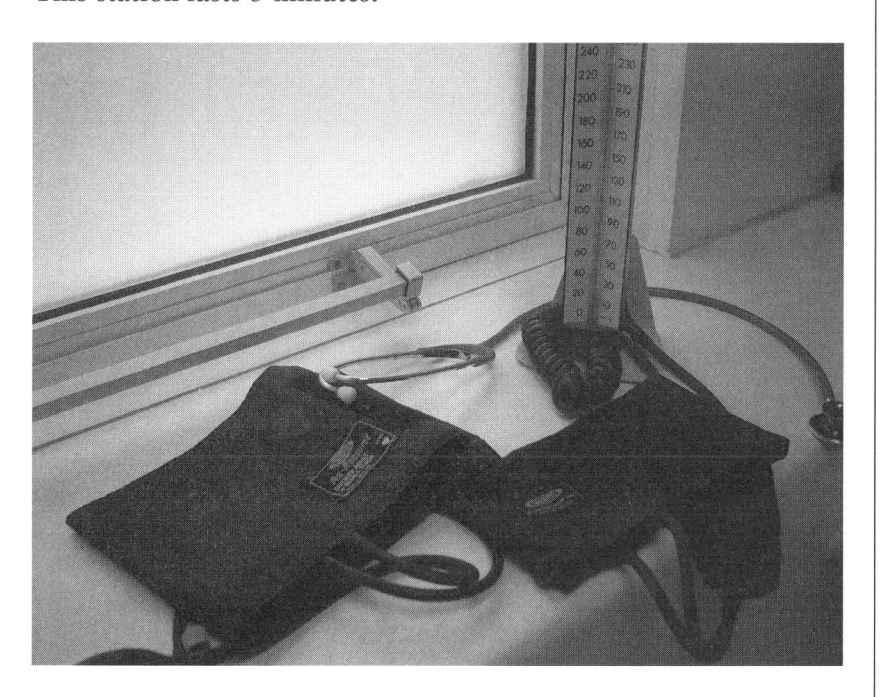

This station lasts 5 minutes.

Station 30
Theme: Mental Test Score

This station tests your ability to obtain a Mental Test Score.

A 70-year-old man is brought in to see you by his wife who suspects he has early Alzheimer's dementia. He has been restless, forgetful and irritable and now has difficulty with speech.

Obtain a Mental Test Score.

This station lasts 5 minutes.

Station 31
Theme: Performing a PV examination

This station tests your ability to perform a per vagina (PV) examination.

A 20-year-old woman presents to you in Casualty complaining of pain on intercourse and profuse foul-smelling vaginal discharge.

Perform a PV examination on the manikin.

This station lasts 5 minutes.

Station 32
Theme: Interpreting an electrocardiogram

This station tests your ability to interpret accurately a 12-lead electrocardiogram.

A 68-year-old woman complains of weight loss and anxiety. You feel her pulse, which is very rapid.

Interpret her 12-lead electrocardiogram. What are the rate, rhythm and diagnosis?

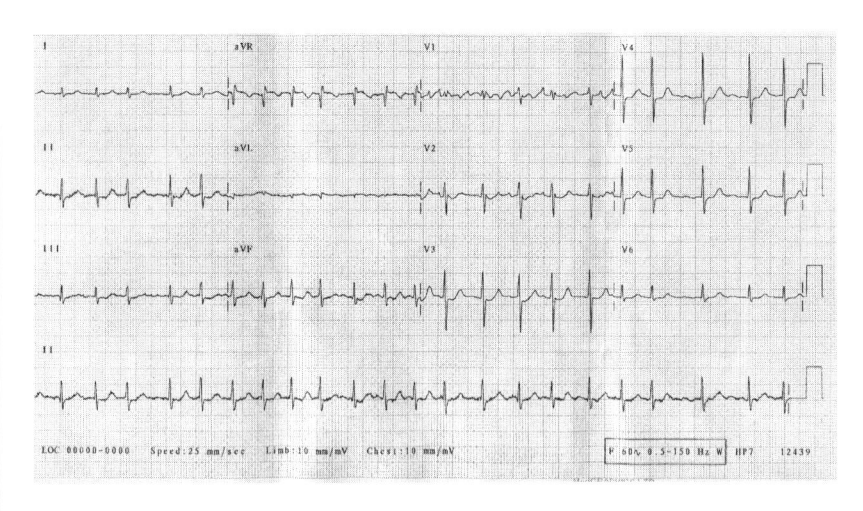

This station lasts 5 minutes.

Station 33
Theme: Glasgow Coma Scale

This station tests your knowledge of and ability to apply the Glasgow Coma Scale.

A 16-year-old schoolboy is struck on the side of the head with a cricket ball. He presents to you in Casualty with a diminished level of consciousness.

Assess his level of consciousness using the Glasgow Coma Scale.

This station lasts 5 minutes.

Station 34
Theme: Interpreting an electrocardiogram

This station tests your ability to interpret accurately a 12-lead electrocardiogram.

A 60-year-old man presents to you with a slow pulse rate. His blood pressure is 130/70.

Interpret his 12-lead electrocardiogram. Give three abnormal findings.

This station lasts 5 minutes.

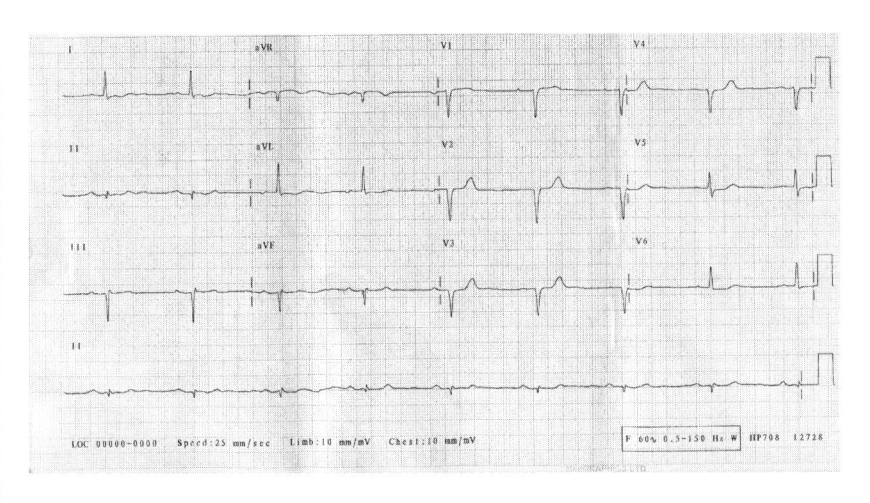

Station 35
Theme: Interpretation of a chest X-ray

This station tests your ability to interpret a chest X-ray.

Master Thomas is a 12-year-old boy who complains of fever, cough and shortness of breath.

Interpret his chest X-ray.

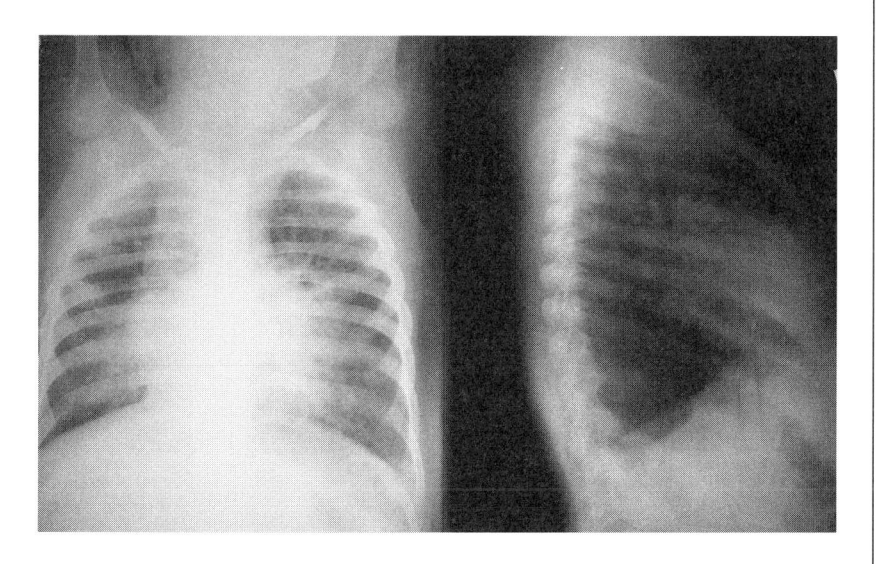

This station lasts 5 minutes.

Station 36
Theme: Fundoscopic examination

This station tests your ability to perform a fundoscopic examination.

Mr Thompson complains of acute onset of headache and pain behind the left eye.

Perform a fundoscopic examination.

This station lasts 5 minutes.

Station 37
Theme: Inserting a cannula into a peripheral vein

This station tests your ability to obtain intravenous access.

Mrs Richards is a 70-year-old woman who presents with absolute dysphagia to solids and liquids. She is emaciated and weak and requires admission for intravenous hydration and investigations.

Demonstrate intravenous cannulation in the manikin.

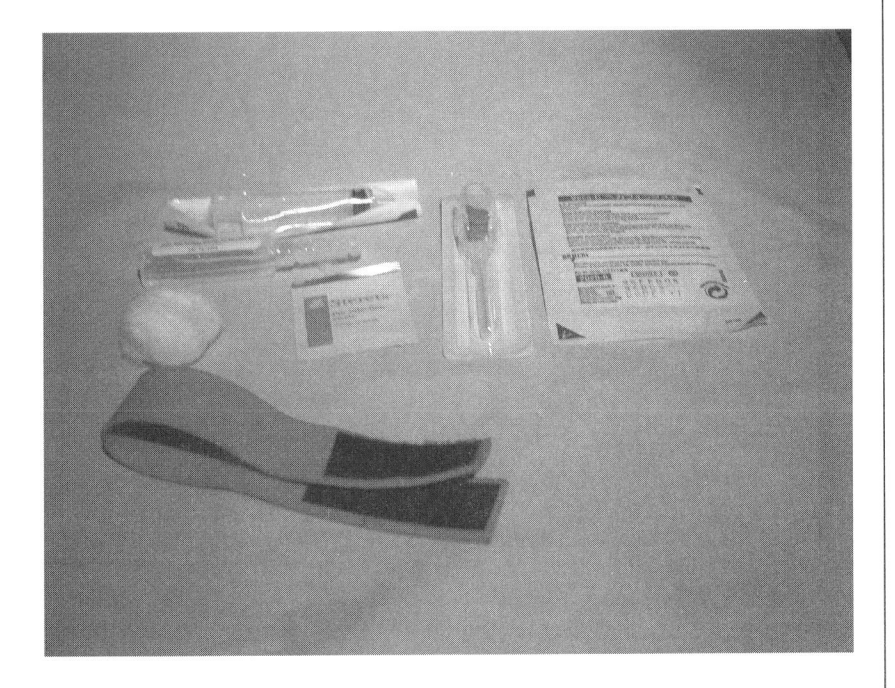

This station lasts 5 minutes.

Station 38
Theme: Examination of the hip

This station tests your ability to perform a hip examination.

Mr Smith is a 60-year-old man who presents to you in the Orthopaedic Outpatient Clinic complaining of increasing left hip pain and stiffness.

Perform a hip examination on Mr Smith (actor).

This station lasts 5 minutes.

Station 39
Theme: Dizziness

This station tests your ability to take a history and reach a diagnosis.

Mr D'Angelo is a 70-year-old man with a history of NIDDM and hypertension. He complains of three episodes of dizziness and vomiting over the past month. The episodes last 6 hours. He denies tinnitus or deafness. He self-stopped taking aspirin 6 months ago. He is on atenolol and gliclazide.

Take a relevant history and suggest a likely diagnosis.

This station lasts 5 minutes.

Station 40
Theme: Interpretation of a chest X-ray

This station tests your ability to interpret a chest X-ray.

Mr Lim is a 65-year-old man who complains of weight loss and persistent cough. On examination, you also note ptosis, miosis, enophthalmos and unilateral anhydrosis.

Interpret his chest X-ray.

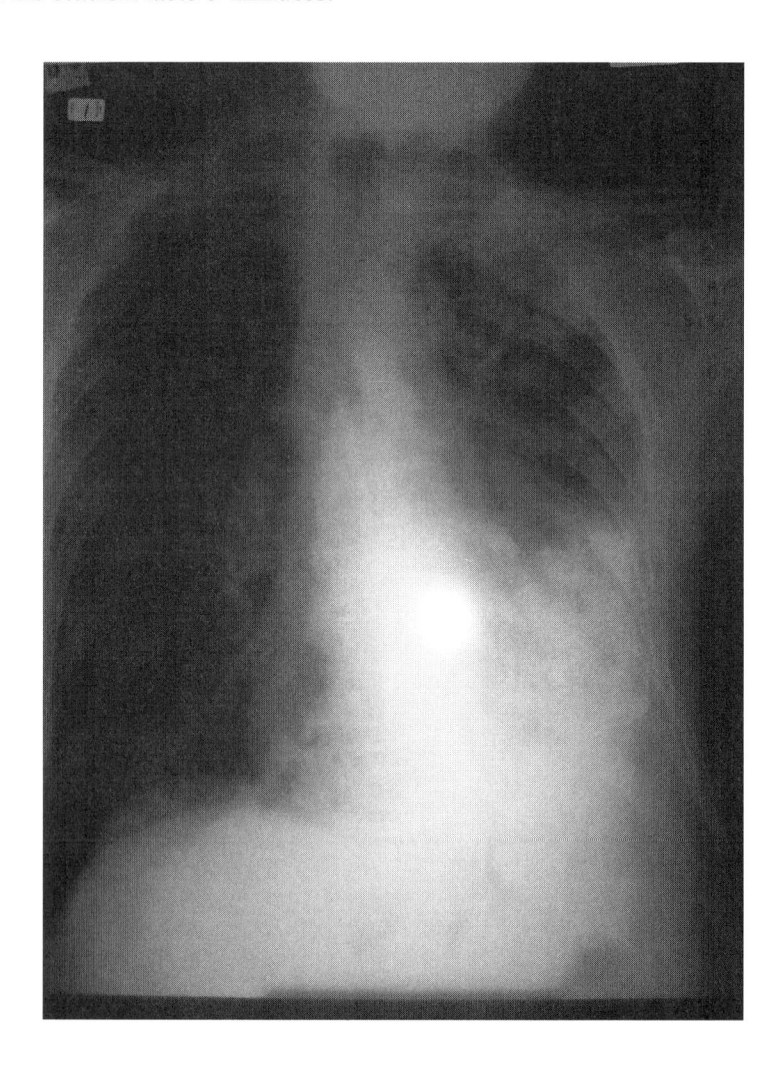

This station lasts 5 minutes.

Station 41
Theme: Wheeze

This station tests your ability to take a history and reach a diagnosis.

Miss Franklin is a 15-year-old girl who complains of wheezing and shortness of breath. It is worse in the winter months and during exercise. She has been sleeping poorly and has required three pillows. She also has a persistent non-productive cough. She has no pets. She does not smoke.

Take a relevant history and suggest a likely diagnosis.

This station lasts 5 minutes.

Station 42
Theme: Duties of a doctor

This station tests your knowledge of the major legal and ethical principles set out in *Duties of a Doctor* published by the General Medical Council (GMC).

Discuss with the examiner your understanding of the principles set out in *Duties of a Doctor*. There are 14 principles in total.

This station lasts 5 minutes.

Station 43
Theme: Breast examination

This station tests your ability to perform a breast examination.

Miss Riley is a 28-year-old woman who complains of a lump in her right breast. She is anxious that she may have breast cancer as her mother died of breast cancer in her 40s.

Perform a breast examination on the manikin. Assume Miss Riley has a 2 cm cystic lump on palpation. What would you next do in Outpatient Clinic?

This station lasts 5 minutes.

Station 44
Theme: Consent for a post mortem

This station tests both your manner for breaking bad news and your ability to obtain informed consent.

Mr Barton, a 72-year-old man, is brought to Accident and Emergency short of breath. His respiratory status becomes severely compromised and he is intubated. He arrests shortly afterwards and is pronounced dead within 2 hours of arrival into the hospital. His wife is in attendance. You suspect pulmonary embolism.

Inform Mrs Barton (actor) that her husband has passed away and obtain informed consent from her for a post mortem examination.

This station lasts 5 minutes.

Station 45
Theme: Weight loss

This station tests your ability to take a history and reach a diagnosis.

Miss Clark is an 18-year-old young woman who presents to you with weight loss, amenorrhoea and depression. You are the Psychiatric SHO.

Take a relevant history and suggest a likely diagnosis.

This station lasts 5 minutes.

Station 46
Theme: Examination of the shoulder joint

This station tests your ability to perform an examination of the shoulder joint.

Mr Clarke is a 30-year-old man who complains of pain and stiffness in his left shoulder. He is an avid tennis player.

Demonstrate on the actor how you would examine his shoulder joint.

This station lasts 5 minutes.

Station 47
Theme: Examination of the hand

This station tests your ability to conduct an examination of the hand.

Mrs Jones is a 40-year-old pregnant woman who complains of tingling and numbness in the fingers of her right hand, which are worse at night.

Examine Mrs Jones's (actor) hands and suggest a likely diagnosis.

This station lasts 5 minutes.

Station 48
Theme: Headache

This station tests your ability to take a relevant history and to reach a diagnosis.

Miss Choi is a 26-year-old woman who complains of generalized headache lasting for several hours. She was started on Microgynon 2 months ago. She states that the headaches are preceded by sensitivity to light and feelings of intense nausea.

Take a relevant history and suggest a likely diagnosis.

This station lasts 5 minutes.

Station 49
Theme: Giving intravenous injections

This station tests your ability to administer an intravenous injection.

Miss Mitchell is a 50-year-old woman with breast cancer who is due for chemotherapy. You are instructed to give her a premed of 8 mg ondansetron iv.

Demonstrate how you would administer ondansetron iv on the manikin.

This station lasts 5 minutes.

Station 50
Theme: Interpretation of a chest X-ray

This station tests your ability to interpret a chest X-ray.

Mrs Khan is a 55-year-old woman who complains of persistent cough and weight loss.

Interpret her chest X-ray.

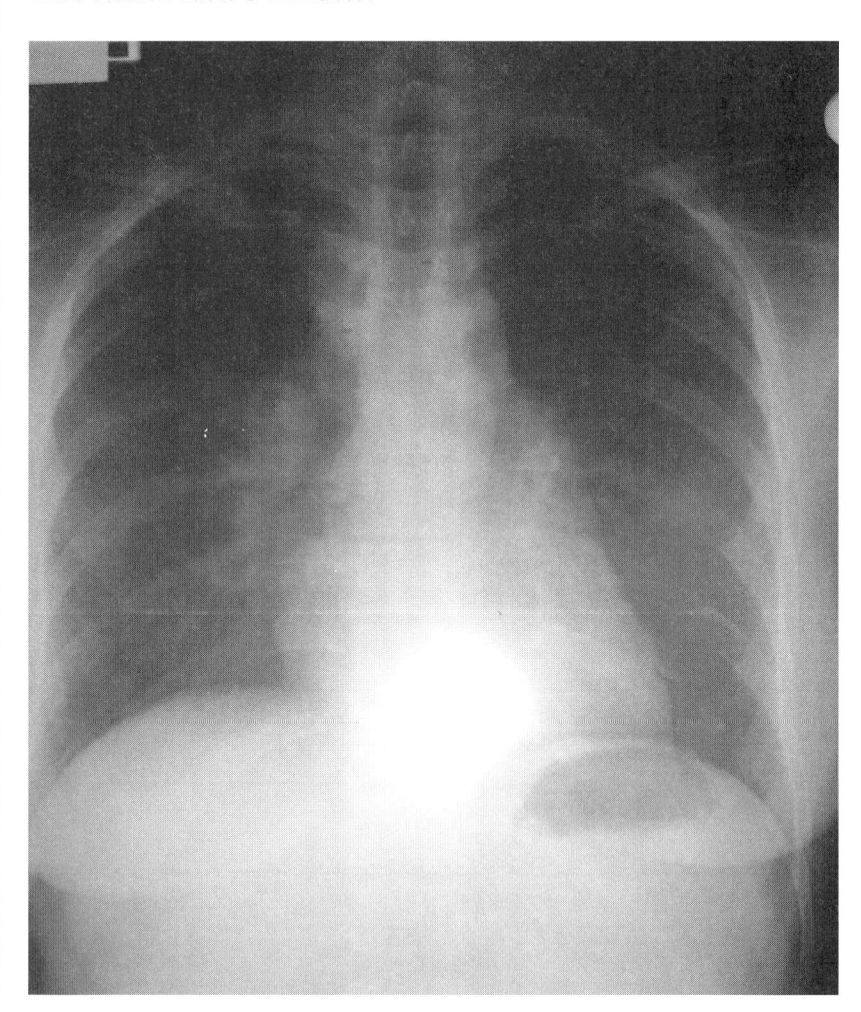

This station lasts 5 minutes.

Station 51
Theme: Administration of an intramuscular injection

This station tests your ability to competently administer an intramuscular injection.

Miss Wharton is a 23-year-old woman who is brought to Accident and Emergency by ambulance in anaphylactic shock. Her companion explains that there were nuts in her salad. She suffers from several food allergies. On examination, she is wearing a facemask with oxygen, her blood pressure is 90/50 and her pulse is 110. She is distressed and dyspnoeic. On examination, both her lips and uvula are markedly swollen.

Which medication does Miss Wharton need urgently and how would you administer it? Demonstrate this on the manikin.

This station lasts 5 minutes.

Station 52
Theme: Palpitations

This station tests your ability to take a history and make a diagnosis.

Mr Park is a 65-year-old man who presents to the Cardiac Outpatient Clinic with a history of palpitations, which last for 5 minutes. He also has associated tightness in the chest, diaphoresis, nausea and faintness. He takes aspirin od and GTN spray as required for his angina.

Take a relevant history and suggest a likely diagnosis.

This station lasts 5 minutes.

Station 53
Theme: Cardiovascular examination

This station tests your ability to conduct a satisfactory cardiovascular examination.

Mrs Collins is a 60-year-old woman who is being admitted for a coronary artery bypass graft operation.

Conduct a cardiovascular examination on Mrs Collins (actor).

This station lasts 5 minutes.

Station 54
Theme: Seeking informed consent for appendicectomy

Miss Cardoza is a 16-year-old girl who was brought to Casualty with acute appendicitis. You are the Surgical SHO on duty and have admitted her with the view to perform an appendicectomy on the emergency theatre list.

Obtain an informed consent from Miss Cardoza for the proposed appendicectomy.

This station lasts 5 minutes.

Station 55
Theme: Administration of oxygen therapy

This station tests your ability to assess competently a patient's airway and administer oxygen therapy safely.

Mr Campbell is a 70-year-old man who is brought to Casualty in respiratory distress. He has a history of chronic obstructive airway disease.

Control the airway and administer oxygen therapy on the manikin.

This station lasts 5 minutes.

Station 56
Theme: Rectal examination

This station tests your ability to perform a rectal examination.

Mr Ling is a 60-year-old man who complains of urinary frequency, dribbling and incontinence for several months. On abdominal examination, his bladder is full and tense. You suspect benign prostatic hypertrophy but at this stage cannot exclude anything sinister.

Demonstrate a rectal examination on the manikin.

This station lasts 5 minutes.

Station 57
Theme: Examination of the chest

This station tests your ability to perform a competent chest examination.

Mr Whittam is a 65-year-old man with chronic obstructive airway disease. He has a 40-pack-year history.

Examine Mr Whittam's (actor) chest.

This station lasts 5 minutes.

Station 58
Theme: Diarrhoea

This station tests your ability to take a history and reach a likely diagnosis.

Mrs Jacobs is a 80-year-old resident of a nursing home who has been referred to you for several episodes of diarrhoea.

Take a history and suggest a likely diagnosis.

This station lasts 5 minutes.

Station 59
Theme: Dysphagia

This station tests your ability to take a pertinent history and reach a diagnosis.

Mrs Stines is a 70-year-old woman who complains of difficulty swallowing food. She also complains of regurgitating food, halitosis and a lump in her throat.

Take a relevant history and suggest a likely diagnosis.

This station lasts 5 minutes.

Station 60
Theme: Emergency management of an acute abdomen

This station tests your ability to manage an acute abdomen.

You are the Medical SHO on duty and have been bleeped by the ward nurse. She explains on the telephone that Mr Simpson, a 55-year-old man, who was admitted 2 days ago with acute myocardial infarction, had just had his supper when he started vomiting and complaining of severe colicky abdominal pain. His temperature is now 38°C, with a blood pressure of 90/60 and pulse rate of 120.

How would you respond?

This station lasts 5 minutes.

Station 61
Theme: Facial nerve palsy

This station tests your ability to conduct an examination of the cranial nerves.

Miss Aglionby is a 26-year-old woman who complains of sudden onset of paralysis of the left side of her face. She denies any hearing loss or the presence of any skin vesicles.

Examine Miss Aglionby's (actor) cranial nerves.

This station lasts 5 minutes.

Station 62
Theme: Interpretation of a chest X-ray

This station tests your ability to interpret a chest X-ray.

Mrs Hobbs is a 68-year-old woman who underwent a mastectomy and now complains of difficulty breathing.

Interpret her chest X-ray.

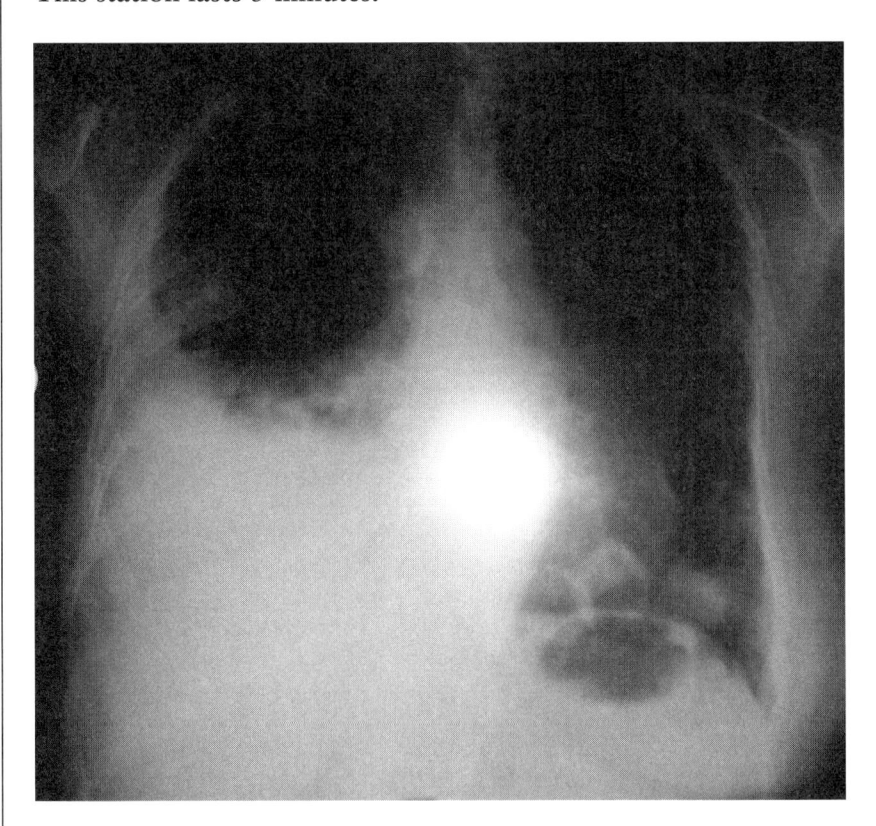

This station lasts 5 minutes.

Station 63
Theme: Examination of the back

This station tests your ability to perform a competent examination of the back.

Mr Oakley is a 55-year-old man who complains of severe lower back pain radiating down his buttocks and calves. He had been lifting heavy boxes the day before.

You suspect sciatica. Examine Mr Oakley's (actor) back.

This station lasts 5 minutes.

Station 64
Theme: Arterial examination of the lower limbs

This station tests your ability to perform a competent arterial examination of the lower limbs.

Mr Wright is a 72-year-old man who complains of pain in his calves after walking short distances. The pain is relieved at rest. He has smoked a pack of cigarettes a day for the past 40 years.

You suspect intermittent claudication. Perform an arterial examination of Mr Wright's (actor) lower limbs.

This station lasts 5 minutes.

Station 65
Theme: Examination of the venous circulation of the lower limbs

This station tests your ability to perform an examination of the venous circulation of the lower limbs.

Mrs Weir is a 55-year-old woman who complains of aching varicose veins at the end of the day, night cramps, a leg ulcer and swelling of the ankles.

You suspect abnormalities with her venous circulation or calf pump failure. Perform an examination of the venous circulation of Mrs Weir's (actor) lower limbs. Attempt to determine whether she has long or short saphenous vein incompetence.

This station lasts 5 minutes.

Station 66
Theme: Examination of a diabetic foot

This station tests your ability to competently examine a diabetic foot.

Mr Cook is a 67-year-old man with IDDM who complains of numbness and burning in his feet, which are worse at night.

Examine Mr Cook's (actor) foot. Remark on any positive findings.

This station lasts 5 minutes.

Station 67
Theme: Neurological examination of the lower limbs

This station tests your ability to perform a competent neurological examination of the lower limbs.

Miss Richardson is a 40-year-old woman who complains of weakness in her legs and blurry vision.

You suspect multiple sclerosis. Conduct a neurological examination of Miss Richardson's (actor) legs.

This station lasts 5 minutes.

Station 68
Theme: Peak flow meter

This station tests your ability to instruct a patient on the use of a peak flow meter and to interpret the results of peak expiratory flow rate.

Miss Carlton is a 22-year-old woman with asthma for which she takes regular salbutamol and ventolin inhalers. She has recently developed a chest infection.

You decide to check her peak expiratory flow rate. Instruct the patient on how to use the peak flow meter and interpret the result.

This station lasts 5 minutes.

Station 69
Theme: Interpretation of a chest X-ray

This station tests your ability to interpret a chest X-ray.

Mr Patel is a 24-year-old man who complains of persistent cough and fever.

Interpret his chest X-ray.

This station lasts 5 minutes.

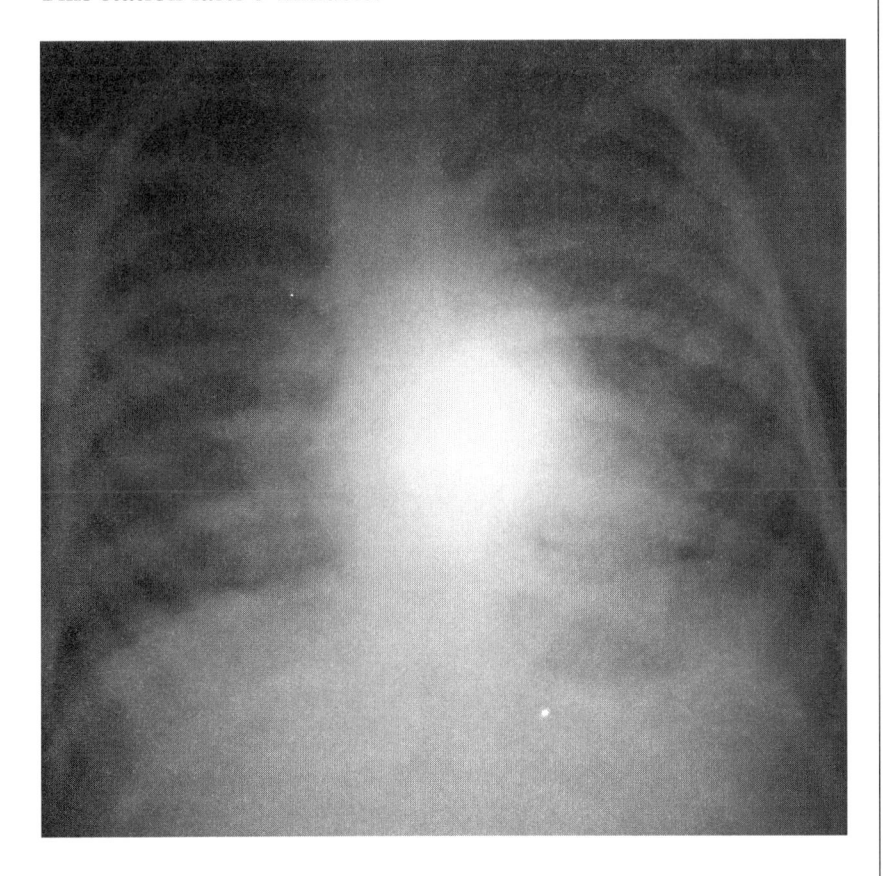

Station 70
Theme: Interpretation of a chest X-ray

This station tests your ability to interpret a chest X-ray.

Mrs Hart is a 40-year-old woman who has arrived off a long-haul flight from Los Angeles. She has been brought to Casualty with difficulty breathing.

Interpret her chest X-ray.

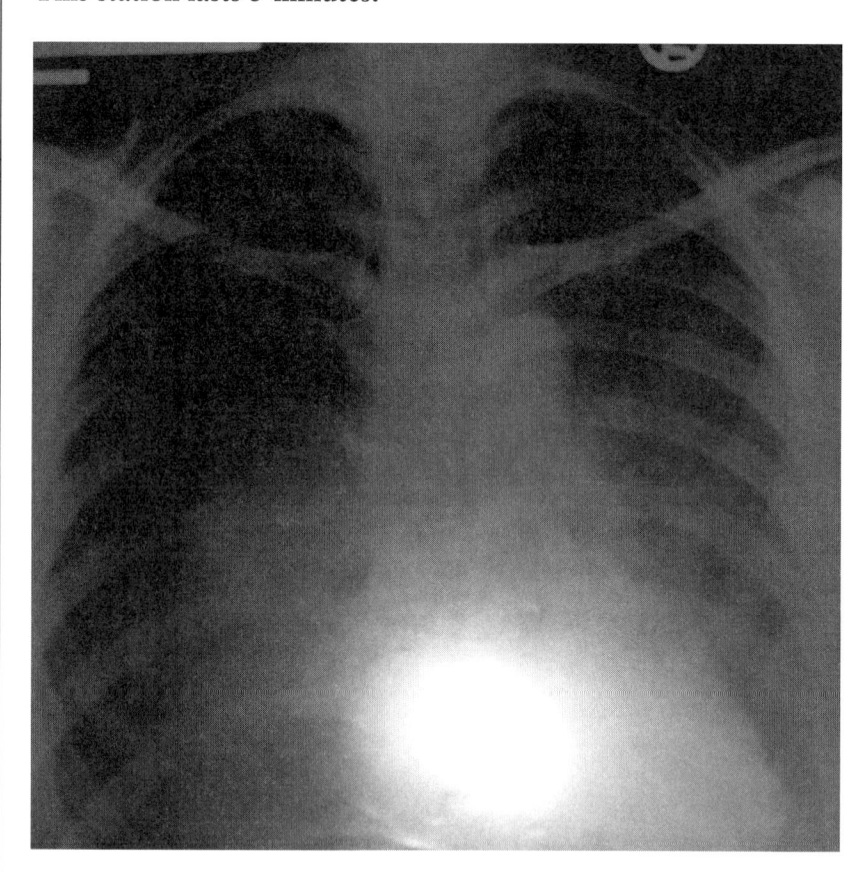

This station lasts 5 minutes.

Station 71
Theme: Diabetic eye

This station tests your ability to perform a fundoscopic examination and reach a diagnosis.

Mr Stanton is a 65-year-old IDDM who has come for his annual eye check-up.

Perform a fundoscopic examination on the manikin and explain your findings.

This station lasts 5 minutes.

Station 72
Theme: Interpretation of a chest X-ray

This station tests your ability to interpret a chest X-ray.

Mr Mills is a 45-year-old homeless man who was found unconscious on the street. He smells of alcohol. He is brought in by ambulance.

Interpret his chest X-ray.

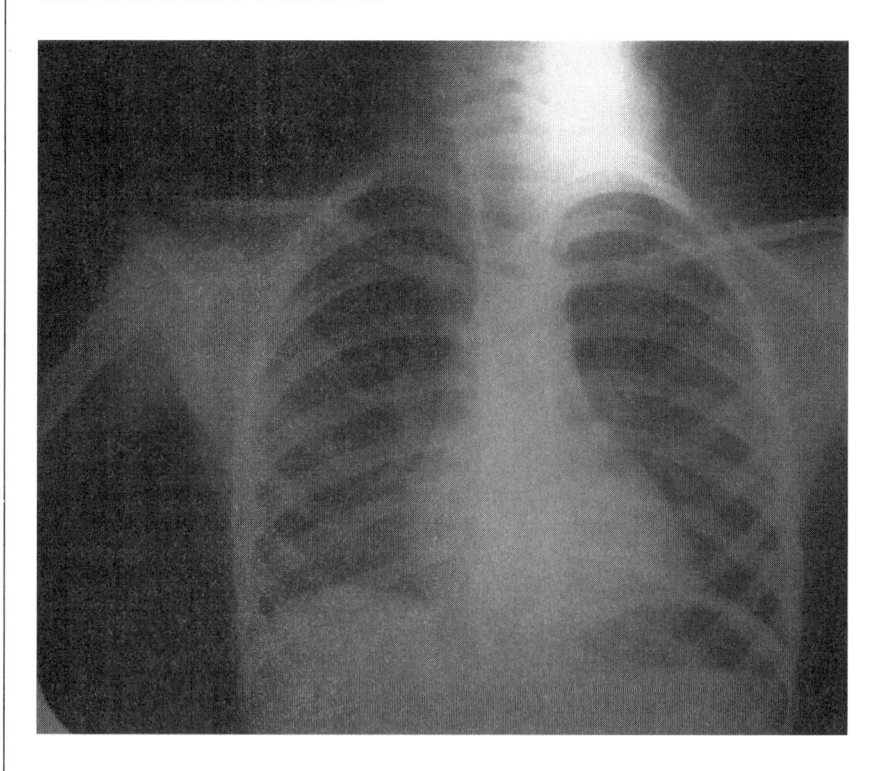

This station lasts 5 minutes.

Station 73
Theme: Neonatal resuscitation

This station tests your knowledge of neonatal resuscitation.

You are the Paediatric SHO on duty and have been summoned to the delivery theatre. A term baby has been handed over to you. She is cyanotic with a heart rate of 90 bpm.

Demonstrate how you would resuscitate the baby on the manikin.

This station lasts 5 minutes.

Station 74
Theme: Abdominal pain

This station tests your ability to take a history and reach a diagnosis.

Mrs White is a 45-year-old obese woman who presents with epigastric pain, fever, nausea and vomiting.

Take a relevant history and suggest a likely diagnosis.

This station lasts 5 minutes.

Station 75
Theme: Fundoscopic examination

This station tests your ability to perform a fundoscopic examination and reach a diagnosis.

Mrs Levitt is a 55-year-old woman who presents to pre-assessment clinic. You note that her blood pressure is 180/100. She is not known to be a hypertensive. She also complains of headaches and nausea. You decide to perform a fundoscopic examination.

Perform a fundoscopic examination on the manikin and explain your findings.

This station lasts 5 minutes.

Station 76
Theme: Discharge instructions post-myocardial infarction

This station tests your ability to communicate with the patient and give sound discharge instructions.

Mr Morris is a 50-year-old man with NIDDM who is being discharged post-myocardial infarction. His discharge medications include glyceryl trinitrate sublingual prn, aspirin od, gliclazide 80 mg od and tenormin 50 mg bd.

Offer Mr Morris (actor) advice upon discharge.

This station lasts 5 minutes.

Station 77
Theme: Discharge instructions for epilepsy

This station tests your ability to communicate and offer sound discharge instructions for epilepsy.

Miss Fields is a 22-year-old woman who has recently been diagnosed with epilepsy. She is discharged home on phenytoin.

Offer Miss Fields (actor) discharge instructions for epilepsy.

This station lasts 5 minutes.

Station 78
Theme: Episodes of loss of consciousness

This station tests your ability to take a relevant history and reach a diagnosis.

Miss Jones is a 20-year-old woman who complains of episodes of loss of consciousness.

Take a relevant history and suggest a likely diagnosis.

This station lasts 5 minutes.

Station 79
Theme: Post-natal depression

This station tests your ability to take a relevant history and offer management.

Mrs Campbell is a 35-year-old woman who delivered a baby boy 3 months ago. She is brought to Casualty by her husband and is tearful, depressed and has rejected her baby.

You are the Psychiatric SHO on duty. Take a history and offer appropriate management.

This station lasts 5 minutes.

Station 80
Theme: Secondary survey

This station tests your knowledge and ability to perform a secondary survey in a resuscitation scenario.

Mr Hewitt is a 40-year-old man who is brought in to Casualty by ambulance after falling out of a second-story window onto a concrete pavement.

Assume the primary survey has been completed. Perform a secondary survey on the manikin.

This station lasts 5 minutes.

Station 81
Theme: Postoperative collapse

This station tests your ability to manage postoperative collapse and give a telephone report.

Mrs Moore is a 50-year-old woman who has undergone oesophagogastrectomy for oesophageal carcinoma. You are the Surgical SHO on duty and are summoned to the ward as her blood pressure is noted to be 90/50 and her pulse rate is 100. She is hooked up to patient-controlled analgesia (PCA). On arrival, you find her drowsy.

Give a telephone report of your management of this patient to the consultant in charge. Address the examiner.

This station lasts 5 minutes.

Station 82
Theme: Telephone advice on meningitis

This station tests your ability to give sound telephone advice on meningitis.

Mrs James is a 35-year-old mother who is telephoning for advice on how to manage her 2-year-old daughter who is febrile with an ear infection.

She is reluctant to bring her daughter into hospital for examination. Give her telephone advice as to why she should bring her daughter to hospital and explain the daughter's risk of meningitis.

This station lasts 5 minutes.

Station 83
Theme: Insomnia

This station tests your ability to take a sympathetic history and suggest management.

Mrs Wesley is a 72-year-old woman who has just lost her husband to metastatic prostate carcinoma. She has not been sleeping well and is depressed.

Take a sympathetic history and suggest suitable management.

This station lasts 5 minutes.

Station 84
Theme: Fever

This station tests your ability to take a history and offer a differential diagnosis for fever.

Mr Akintillo is a 25-year-old African man who presents with fever, which has lasted for 1 week.

Take a relevant history and offer a differential diagnosis for the fever.

This station lasts 5 minutes.

Station 85
Theme: Myocardial infarction

This station tests your ability to manage a patient with acute myocardial infarction.

Mr Patel is a 65-year-old man who is brought to Casualty by ambulance suffering from severe chest pain radiating down his left arm, which is unrelieved by glyceryl trinitrate sublingual tablets. He has a history of angina.

You are the Casualty SHO on duty. Explain to the examiner how you would manage the patient.

This station lasts 5 minutes.

Station 86
Theme: Writing-up findings from a physical exam

This station tests your ability to maintain effective records through the writing-up of findings from a physical examination.

Mr Wilson is a 45-year-old man who presents with weakness in both legs. He states that the sensation in his legs is normal.

Perform a neurological examination on Mr Wilson (actor) and write-up your findings. Omit the test of sensation for the sake of time.

This station lasts 5 minutes.

Station 87
Theme: Initial trauma assessment

This station tests your knowledge and ability to perform an initial trauma assessment.

Miss Hamilton is a 24-year-old woman who is brought to Casualty by ambulance having been involved in a road traffic accident. The paramedics report that she is a victim of a hit and run. She was struck on her right side and flung 20 feet across the road by a speeding vehicle.

Perform an initial trauma assessment on the manikin.

This station lasts 5 minutes.

Station 88
Theme: Examination of the neck

This station tests your ability to examine the neck.

Mrs Bailey is a 56-year-old woman who presents with a mass in the neck that she has had for 6 months.

You are the ENT SHO on duty. Examine Mrs Bailey's (actor) neck.

This station lasts 5 minutes.

Station 89
Theme: Writing-up findings from a physical examination

This station tests your ability to maintain effective records through the writing-up of findings from a physical examination.

Mr Jamieson is a 55-year-old man with chronic hypercarbia (COAD).

Examiner Mr Jamieson's (actor) chest and write-up your findings.

This station lasts 5 minutes.

Station 90
Theme: Interpretation of results

This station tests your ability to interpret correctly results and reach a diagnosis.

A 46-year-old man is referred to the Hypertension Clinic. His BP is 172/112 with a pulse rate of 72 bpm regular. He complains of generalized weakness, occasional muscle cramps, thirst and polyuria. He is not taking diuretics, steroids, laxatives or maxolon.

Study the results of the investigations below and suggest a likely diagnosis. How would you confirm this diagnosis?

This station lasts 5 minutes.

- Haemoglobin: 11.4 g dl^{-1}
- White cell count: 5.6×10^9 l^{-1}
- Platelets: 146×10^9 l^{-1}
- Sodium: 148 mmol l^{-1}

- Potassium: 2.4 mmol l^{-1}
- Bicarbonate: 34 mmol l^{-1}
- Urea: 5.0 mmol l^{-1}
- Creatinine: 110 µmol l^{-1}
- Glucose: 6.0 mmol l^{-1}

- Urinanalysis: normal

- Twenty-four-hour urinary potassium excretion: 60 mmol

- CXR: normal
- ECG: rate of 70 bpm, regular sinus rhythm, flattened T-waves in all leads
- Renal ultrasound: normal
- Renal venography: normal

Station 91
Theme: Interpretation of blood results

This station tests your ability to interpret correctly blood results and reach a diagnosis.

Miss Smythson is a 20-year-old woman who complains of malaise and easy bruisability. She is always covered in bruises. Her gums bleed when she brushes her teeth, and her periods are heavy and painful. She also complains of recurrent painful mouth ulcers. She has no family history of bleeding dyscrasias. She does not smoke or drink. She is not taking any medication. On examination, you note gum hypertrophy, oral candidiasis and painful lymphadenopathy.

You decide to take blood for full blood count, clotting, and urea and electrolytes. The results have come back. Interpret the results below and suggest a likely diagnosis. How would you confirm this diagnosis?

This station lasts 5 minutes.

- White cell count: 11.8×10^9 l^{-1}
- Blood film: few immature blast cells
- Haemoglobin: 6.5 g dl^{-1}
- Mean cell volume: 84 fl
- Platelets: 10×10^9 l^{-1}
- ESR: 20 mm h^{-1}

- INR: 0.9
- APTT: 1.1

- Sodium: 139 mmol l^{-1}
- Potassium: 4.6 mmol l^{-1}
- Urea: 6.7 mmol l^{-1}
- Creatinine: 116 μmol l^{-1}
- Glucose: 5.0 mmol l^{-1}

Station 92
Theme: Fundoscopic examination

This station tests your ability to perform a fundoscopic examination and reach a diagnosis.

Mr Daya is a 24-year-old motorcyclist who was hit by a turning vehicle and flung off his motorbike. He was not wearing a helmet. His initial vital signs are BP 140/90, pulse 90 bpm and respiratory rate of 25 breaths per minute. He is brought to Casualty by ambulance. On arrival, his vital signs are BP is 170/100, pulse rate is 60 bpm, with irregular respirations. He is agitated and drowsy.

Perform a fundoscopic examination on the manikin. Remark on your findings and suggest the most likely cause.

This station lasts 5 minutes.

Station 93
Theme: Consent for inguinal herniorrhaphy

This station tests your ability to take consent for inguinal herniorrhaphy.

Mr Jacobs is a 60-year-old man with a right indirect inguinal hernia. He has a history of angina, CVA and hypertension. You are the Surgical SHO in the pre-assessment clinic.

Take consent from Mr Jacobs for a right hernia repair operation. Suggest the most suitable technique for him.

This station lasts 5 minutes.

Station 94
Theme: Terminal care

This station tests your ability to discuss terminal care with a patient's relative.

Mrs Khan has come to you to discuss terminal care for her husband who has terminal metastatic lung carcinoma. She would like him to die in a dignified manner at home with his family present.

Discuss terminal care with Mrs Khan (actor).

This station lasts 5 minutes.

Station 95
Theme: Fundoscopic examination

This station tests your ability to perform a fundoscopic examination and reach a diagnosis.

Mr Kane is a 67-year-old man who has been referred by his optician for findings on his fundi.

Examine his fundi and comment on your findings.

This station lasts 5 minutes.

Station 96
Theme: Anxiety

This station tests your ability to take a history and suggest appropriate management.

Mrs Holland is a 45-year-old woman who complains of difficulty sleeping, anxiety and an increasing number of panic attacks. She describes these occasions as feeling as though she is choking. She cannot breathe, has palpitations, is sweaty and has tingling in her fingers.

You are the Psychiatric SHO. Take a sympathetic history and suggest management.

This station lasts 5 minutes.

Station 97
Theme: Explaining diagnosis and management

This station tests your communication skills.

Mrs Tang is a 30-year-old woman who is 6 weeks pregnant. She presents to Casualty with right-sided abdominal pain and scant per vagina (PV) bleed. On examination, she is extremely tender in the right iliac fossa. On speculum examination, the cervical os is closed and there is a scant bloody discharge. On PV exam, there is no cervical excitation, but she is tender in the right adnexa with a palpable mass. The urinalysis shows no proteins, leukocytes or nitrates. She has 2+ blood.

You are the Gynaecology SHO. Explain to Mrs Tang (actor) that you suspect she may have an ectopic pregnancy. Explain how you plan to manage her.

This station lasts 5 minutes.

Station 98
Theme: Alcoholism

This station tests your ability to take a history on alcohol intake and to give advice on rehabilitation.

Mr Marsland is a 50-year-old man who is being seen in pre-assessment clinic for a hernia operation. His full blood count results show an elevated mean corpuscular volume and his liver function tests reveal an elevated γ-glutamyl-transferase.

You suspect alcoholism. Take a history on the patient's alcohol intake and offer advice on rehabilitation.

This station lasts 5 minutes.

Station 99
Theme: Giving advice on treatment for acne

This station tests your communication skills.

Miss Wood is a 14-year-old girl with widespread acne covering her face, back and arms. She has tried trimethoprim and benzamycin gel with no success.

You are the Dermatology SHO. Suggest to the patient's mother (actor) that her daughter tries triple therapy with minocin MR tablets, dianette pills and differin gel. The mother is anxious to know about any side-effects with these drugs. Counsel her.

This station lasts 5 minutes.

Station 100
Theme: Haematuria

This station tests your ability to take a relevant history and suggest appropriate investigations.

Miss Caine is a 20-year-old woman who presents to Casualty with a 3-day history of right-sided flank pain and macroscopic haematuria. On examination, a large, non-tender, irregular, ballotable mass is palpated at each flank. Her BP is 150/100. Otherwise, her examination is unremarkable. Her serum urea returns as 12 mmol l^{-1} and her creatinine as 160 µmol l^{-1}.

Take a relevant history and suggest appropriate investigations to reach a diagnosis.

This station lasts 5 minutes.

Station 1: Answers

1. Communication

Establish a rapport with the patient:

- Smile, shake hands and introduce yourself to the patient. 'Hello Mr Johnson, my name is Doctor X. Welcome to the Rheumatology Clinic.'
- **You will fail if you forget to introduce yourself to the patient!**

Maintain good eye contact and listen attentively. Respond to verbal and non-verbal cues.

Use appropriate questioning strategies. Avoid medical jargon!

2. Presenting complaint

Elicit a history of acute onset recurrent mono-arthritis:

- 'Tell me more about the joint pain in your left big toe.'
- 'Describe the nature of the pain? Is it constant, intermittent, dull, sharp, etc?'
- 'Does anything make the pain better or worse? Is it worse in the morning?'
- 'Was the toe swollen or the skin red?'
- 'When did you have your first attack?'
- 'Did you have other attacks?'
- 'What painkillers have you tried?'
- 'What has your GP prescribed? Was it successful or not?'
- 'What are your concerns?'

3. Other history

Take a past medical history: pertinent positives include psoriasis, hypothyroidism, hypertension, renal disease and primary hyperparathyroidism, i.e. causes of hyperuricaemia.

Take a surgical history: a recent history of surgery may precipitate an attack.

Take a drug history: pertinent positives include thiazide diuretics and salicylates.

Take a social history:

- 'What is your occupation?'
- 'Are you married?'
- 'Do you exercise?' Impaired excretion of uric acid is associated with increased lactic acid production from alcohol, exercise and/or starvation.
- 'Do you smoke or drink alcohol? How much alcohol do you drink in one day? Do you drink red wine, port or spirits?'
- Ask about a diet of meat, especially game such as quail, pheasant and grouse, of tomatoes or of other foods high in purine? Excess purine is a contributory factor to hyperuricaemia.

Exclude a history of sexually transmitted diseases (STD), in particular gonococcal arthritis or urethritis?: 'Have you had any extramarital sexual intercourse?'

Exclude symptoms of other joint diseases:

- 'Any other joints affected – ankles, knees?'
- Bear in mind that gout may also affect these lower limb joints.
- Exclude Reiter's syndrome, osteoarthritis, etc.

4. Diagnosis (at the 30-second bell)

The patient's history most likely suggests a diagnosis of gout. On clinical examination, I would check his blood pressure, weight (BMI) and look, in particular, for signs of tophi in the ear lobe. I would confirm the diagnosis upon aspiration of synovial fluid from the affected joint and finding needle-shaped, negatively birefringent crystals under the microscope. I would check his serum uric acid but understand its limitations with its high false-positive and -negative results. I would manage the patient conservatively with advice about weight reduction, reduction in alcohol consumption, avoidance of foods high in purine and avoidance of salicylates, and suggest good fluid intake to avoid dehydration especially after exercise. I would suggest indocin at 50 mg 0 tds to manage acute attacks of gout with promising results within 24–48 hours.

Note that the above answer contains more than adequate material to obtain a grade of A or excellent for this single station.

Station 2: Answers

1. Communication

Establish a rapport with the patient. Smile and introduce yourself. Reassure the patient that even though she is under 16, the law states that she is still entitled to emergency contraception without the knowledge or consent of her parents and that everything that is said between the two of you remains strictly confidential. Ensure she is Gillick competent.

Maintain good eye contact and listen attentively.

Use appropriate questioning strategies.

2. Presenting complaint

Elicit a history confirming unprotected sex and risk of pregnancy:

- 'Why do you think you could be pregnant?'
- 'Did vaginal penetration occur?'
- 'What form of contraception had you been using? Why do you think it has failed?'
- Confirm the potential barrier method or pill failure.
- 'Where in your menstrual cycle are you?' The most fertile period is days 10–19.
- 'What are your views on regular contraception?'

3. Other history

Take a gynaecology history:

- 'When did you start menstruating?'
- 'Are your periods regular? How long do they last? Are they heavy?'
- 'Have you ever been treated for sexually transmitted diseases (STD)?'
- 'Have you ever been pregnant before?'

Take a drug history: 'Are you taking any antibiotics or any other medication?' The combined oral contraceptive pill is less effective in the presence of oral antibiotics or anti-epileptic drugs.

4. Management (at the 30-second bell)

I would inform her that she has two options. She can take Levonelle–2 (one tablet now and one in 12 hours), which in her particular case gives her an 85% rate of successful emergency contraception, or be fitted with an IUD coil, which would be '99% effective.' Each tablet contains 750 mcg levonorgestrel (progestogen only). According to the Faculty of Family Planning April 2000 Guidance Sheet for Emergency Contraception and the Recommendation for Clinical Practice, Levonelle–2 is 95% effective if taken within 24 hours of unprotected sex. This drops to 85% at 48 hours and 58% at 72 hours. If she would like a method that is 99% effective, an intrauterine coil can be fitted. This method of emergency contraception is effective up to 5 days following unprotected sex.

Station 3: Answers

You will be asked to interpret at least one 12-lead electrocardiogram in the OSCE!

1. This is a normal electrocardiogram (ECG).
2. The rate is 75.
3. The rhythm is normal sinus.
4. The axis is normal. A quick guide to determining the axis is to look at leads I–III. If the main deflection in leads I and II are the R waves and the QRS complex in lead III is of zero magnitude (equal positive and negative deflections), the axis is normal.
5. The P wave is normal. The P–R interval is normal. The QRS complexes are normal.
6. There are no obvious abnormalities.

Station 4: Answers

1. Communication

Introduce yourself to the patient.

2. Presenting complaint

'When was your last menstrual period? Could you be pregnant? Or are you currently menstruating?' Confirm pregnancy by a urine HCG test. Urinalysis is also routinely performed with the urine specimen.

If positive, be suspicious of a diagnosis of miscarriage versus ectopic pregnancy:

- 'Do you have pain? Where does it hurt?' Unilateral iliac fossa pain may arouse suspicion of an ectopic pregnancy but can also arise from a corpus luteum cyst, i.e. the ovary that released the egg in normal pregnancy.
- 'When did the bleeding begin? Have you passed any clots? Any foetal material?' Try to gauge the amount of blood loss and whether she has completed a miscarriage.
- 'Have you ever had a scan for this pregnancy?' A previous scan confirming intrauterine pregnancy can reassure you that you are not dealing with an ectopic pregnancy.

If negative, ask questions geared towards narrowing the following list of possibilities. The UK 'sieve' for assessing the aetiology of any medical or surgical disorder is as follows:

- Congenital: bicornuate uterus
- Infective: pelvic inflammatory disease (PID)
- Inflammatory
- Neoplastic: fibroids, endometrial polyps, endometrial or cervical neoplasm
- Traumatic: perforation of the uterus secondary to IUD insertion
- Metabolic: hypothyroidism is associated with menorrhagia
- Iatrogenic: anticoagulants
- Idiopathic
- Others: adenomyosis, normal variant

3. Other history

Take an obstetric history:
- Gravida is the number of times a woman has been pregnant.
- Para is the number of live and still births after 24 weeks.
- Are there any previous miscarriages or ectopic pregnancies?
- Any history of ante- or postpartum haemorrhage?

Take a gynaecology history: does she have regular menstrual cycles? What are the lengths of cycles in days? Are there heavy or light periods?

When was her last cervical smear? Was it normal or abnormal? She should be summoned for a routine cervical smear every 3 years during childbearing years.

What does she use for contraception? Has she recently been fitted with a coil (IUD)?

Does she have a regular partner? Is there a history of sexually transmitted diseases (STD)?

Take a drug history: is she taking warfarin or aspirin?

Take a pertinent past medical and surgical history: does she suffer from thyroid disease?

4. Diagnosis (at the 30-second bell)

If the patient is pregnant, a diagnosis of an ectopic pregnancy versus miscarriage is likely. A patient with a ruptured ectopic pregnancy may present in hypovolaemic shock with signs of peritonism. This patient should be resuscitated immediately and taken to theatre by the gynaecology team on call.

If the patient is stable, a transvaginal ultrasound will help differentiate between an ectopic pregnancy and a miscarriage that is complete or incomplete. Blood tests for serum β-HCG and progesterone may also be used to determine whether the pregnancy is viable or not. A progesterone level of < 40 is indicative of the latter. If the miscarriage is incomplete, i.e. visualization of retained products of conception on the ultrasound, the patient should be offered evacuation of retained products of conception (ERPC), which can usually be performed as a day case.

If the patient is not pregnant and the bleeding is one of menorrhagia, further investigations may be required to make a diagnosis.

Investigations should include full blood count, thyroid function tests, transvaginal ultrasound and endometrial biopsy (if the patient is > 40 years of age). Acute arrest for heavy bleeding can be achieved with norethisterone (a high dose of progesterone). Long-term management may include combined oral contraceptive pills and/or the use of antifibrinolytic agents such as tranexamic acid 1.0–1.5 g o tds or qds during the heavy days of the cycle.

Station 5: Answers

1. Communication

2. Presenting complaint

Elicit a history of acute otitis externa: 'When did the ear pain begin? Is it associated with ear discharge? Have you been abroad recently? Have you been swimming? Do you use cotton buds to clean your ears? Have you had your ears syringed for wax build-up recently?'

Alternatively, ask questions to exclude otitis media: 'Do you have a temperature? Have you had a recent cold? Is your hearing diminished?' Is this of an acute nature or recurrent?

Other causes include herpes zoster oticus (Ramsay–Hunt syndrome), which is associated with vesicles in the external auditory meatus and is most commonly seen in the elderly population.

Ask questions to exclude causes of referred pain to the ear. Causes of referred otalgia include:

- Arthritis/cervical spondylosis
- Soft tissue injury to the second or third cervical nerves
- Dental disease or temporomandibular joint (TMJ) dysfunction via the trigeminal nerve
- Rhinosinusitis, salivary gland disease, nasopharyngeal disease
- Oropharyngeal infections (tonsillitis, quinsy, pharyngitis, post-tonsillectomy)
- Tumours affecting the glossopharyngeal or vagus nerves

3. Other history

Medical history: diabetics are at risk for malignant otitis externa. Get a history of chickenpox to exclude shingles.

4. Diagnosis

A diagnosis of acute otitis externa is most likely if presented with a patient with a painful, malodorous discharging ear and a history of contaminated water exposure to the ear or irritation of the ear canal with cotton buds. The treatment includes aural toilet, insertion of a Pope wick to keep the canal open if it is oedematous, regular instillation of topical antibiotic ear-drops (sofradex, otosporin, gentisone, etc.) and keeping the ear dry during treatment.

Station 6: Answers

1. Be systematic in your interpretation of the X-ray.

2. Look at the chest X-ray to determine if the view is marked as AP or PA, or whether it is a lateral view of the chest. 'This is a PA view of the chest.'

3. Comment on any obvious abnormality. 'The obvious abnormality on this chest X-ray is the presence of right-middle lobe collapse. This patient has pneumonia.'

4. Plan to review the heart, mediastinum, the diaphragm, lung fields, soft tissues (breasts) and bones.

5. Plan to review the apices, the hila, behind the heart, and the costophrenic angles for any pleural effusions.

6. Remark on the heart and mediastinum. The cardiothoracic ratio is the heart width ratio to the chest width, and this should be < 50%. Remark on cardiomegaly, if present. Remark on a widened mediastinum, if present. This would suggest aortic dissection, thymus, thyroid, lymph nodes or tumour, and a lateral view should be requested. Remark on whether a mass is in the superior, anterior, middle or posterior mediastinum.

7. Remark on the hila, which is composed of pulmonary arteries and veins, lymph nodes and airways. The left hilum is usually 1 cm higher than the right hilum. Remark on enlargement (pulmonary arterial hypertension) or changes in density, which may suggest tumour or lymphadenopathy. Hilar lymphadenopathy may suggest tuberculosis, sarcoidosis, lymphoma or metastases.

8. Check the diaphragm. The right hemidiaphragm is normally 3 cm higher than the left side, and on the lateral view passes through the heart shadow. If the hemidiaphragm is elevated, think subphrenic abscess, phrenic nerve palsy, hepatomegaly, diaphragmatic rupture or loss of lung volume. The costophrenic angles should be sharp. If blunted, think hyperinflation or effusion. Check for free air under the diaphragm in an erect chest X-ray, which suggests peritonitis.

9. Check the root of the neck and trachea. The trachea should be midline. In tension pneumothorax, remark if it is deviated

away from the side of the pneumothorax. Remark on any paratracheal lymphadenopathy.

10. Remark on the lung fields. Increased translucency may occur in the following situations: pneumothorax, bullous changes in emphysema, pulmonary embolus, pulmonary hypertension or hyperinflation in chronic hypercarbia (COAD).

11. Remark on any abnormal opacities: coin lesions (solitary pulmonary nodule), collapse, consolidation, linear opacities, ring shadows (pulmonary oedema, bronchiectasis, abscess, tumour, or cavitating lesions) or diffuse lung shadowing.

12. Attempt to distinguish between nodular, alveolar or reticular shadowing. The causes of nodular shadowing include granulomas, malignancies, mitral stenosis, pneumoconioses, septic emboli and viral pneumonia. Some causes of alveolar shadowing include: alveolar proteinosis, ARDS, drugs, head injury, infection, pulmonary oedema, pulmonary haemorrhage, etc. Some causes of reticular shadowing include auto-immune diseases, asbestosis, cryptogenic fibrosing alveolitis, extrinsic allergic alveolitis, fibrosis (tuberculosis, histoplasma), malignancy, sarcoidosis, silicosis, etc.

13. Remark on the soft tissues for subcutaneous emphysema, absence of breast tissue (mastectomy), etc.

14. Remark on the bones – clavicle, ribs, vertebrae – for the presence of any obvious abnormality or fracture.

Station 7: Answers

1. Politely introduce yourself to the patient.

2. Ask if you may examine his ears.

3. Ask him which is the better hearing ear.

4. Ask him if the ear is tender before you touch it.

5. Sit down alongside the patient and use a light source as you examine the pinna and behind for scars, redness or discharge.

6. Assemble an otoscope or auroscope – whichever is provided – and examine the better hearing ear first unless told only to examine the right ear. Remember to retract the pinna (upwards, outwards and backwards) to straighten the tortuous 2.4 cm external auditory canal.

7. Examine the canal for oedema, discharge and vesicles.

8. Examine the tympanic membrane for perforations. Is the perforation dry or wet, central or marginal (involving the entire eardrum)? What structures can you see through the perforation? Malleus, incudostapedial joint, promontory, etc.

9. Examine the pars flaccida (attic of the tympanic membrane for crusts) and the pars tensa for a bulging membrane or a retracted membrane.

10. At this point, the examiner may ask you what you have found. The diagnosis may be a tympanic membrane perforation, mastoid cavity, otitis media, otitis externa, etc.

11. In reality, a complete ear examination continues with Steps 12–14. However, owing to the time permitted, you will only be judged on your ability to use the auroscope or otoscope confidently and professionally.

12. Conduct free-field speech tests. Rub the tragus of the non-examining ear to occlude the canal. Whisper words to the exposed test ear at distances of 60 cm and then repeat different words at conversational level at 60 cm and then 15 cm from the exposed ear. Repeat different words at a raised voice level

at 60 cm and 15 cm. This will give you an idea of the decibel hearing loss.

13. Conduct the Rinne and Weber tuning fork tests using a 512-kHz fork.

14. For the Weber test, place the vibrating fork on the middle of the patient's forehead and ask him which ear he can hear the fork the loudest or if it sounds the same in both ears? If he cannot hear the fork, place it on the bridge of the nose. The patient should hear the tuning fork better in the left ear if he has a sensorineural hearing loss in the right ear or he should hear the tuning fork better in the right ear if he has a conductive hearing loss of the right ear.

15. For the Rinne test, ask the patient to tell you which is louder? First place the tuning fork on the mastoid process and then hold the vibrating fork 4 cm away from the external auditory meatus and ask him to tell you which is louder. Alternatively, the original test was to wait until the fork could be heard no longer on the mastoid process and asking the patient whether he could then hear any sound when placing the fork in front of the ear. In either case, if sound is better heard when the fork is on the mastoid process, a conductive hearing loss is suggested, i.e. bone conduction is better than air conduction. If the tuning fork is heard louder or continues to be heard after decay of the fork on the mastoid process, then the patient either has normal hearing in that ear or a sensorineural hearing loss.

16. Test the facial nerve. Ask the patient to raise his eyebrows (temporal branch), shut his eyes tightly (zygomatic branch), blow his cheeks (buccal branch) and show you his teeth (mandibular branch).

Station 8: Answers

1. Explain to the examiner that you would introduce yourself to the patient. Do not address the manikin.

2. Explain to the examiner that you would then explain the procedure in layman's terms and give reasons why you suggest this should be done. Select the appropriate sized Foley catheter (12–16 Fr). The size in French gauge correlates with the diameter of the catheter.

3. In uncircumcized men, the foreskin needs to be retracted to prep the glans penis. Assume the manikin is circumcized. Put on a pair of sterile gloves. Remember to use aseptic technique.

4. Clean the manikin's penis with cotton balls or gauze dipped in the antiseptic solution provided times three. Discard the used swabs and drape the manikin's groin with sterile paper towel drapes.

5. Apply sterile lignocaine gel to the tip of the catheter and instil the rest of the gel into the penile urethra.

6. Stretch the penis with your non-dominant hand at right angles to the body and slowly advance the catheter with your dominant hand to the hilt or until urine emerges. Ensure that you are drawing out urine.

7. Check the balloon volume size and inflate the catheter balloon with the appropriate amount of saline as indicated on the catheter instructions. The balloon capacity may not always be 10 ml. Connect the exposed end of the Foley catheter to the drainage bag.

8. Slowly retract the catheter until resistance is felt when the inflated balloon comes to rest at the bladder neck.

9. Tidy up after yourself.

10. Explain that you would thank the patient for his cooperation.

11. You will be marked on how fluent and professional you have conducted yourself.

Station 9: Answers

Guidelines to counselling can be obtained from http://www.jhuccp.org/pr/j48/counsel.stm. These guidelines suggest using the mnemonic 'GATHER'.

1. **Greet** the patient and introduce yourself.

2. **Ask** the patient what her reasons are for opting for tubal sterilization. Ask her about her partner and whether he has considered vasectomy, which is a safer option and can be performed under a local anaesthetic.

3. **Tell** the patient about her alternative options. In the patient's case, as she has had a healthy liver transplant, her liver is no longer diseased and she can take the combined oral contraceptive pill without fear of increased first-pass hepatic metabolism in a diseased liver. Explain that other options include:

   - Implanon is a contraceptive implant that is inserted under the skin of the inner upper arm and lasts for 3 years. It is 99% effective.

   - The Depo-Provera or Noristerat contraceptive injection lasts for 12 and 8 weeks respectively and is 99% effective.

   - IUD (in view of her liver transplant, this form of contraception, i.e. a foreign body in the uterus, may not be her first choice).

   Tell the patient about the risks and benefits of tubal sterilization:

   - It is permanent and consequently there is a risk of regret as she is only 22 and may not be ready for permanent sterilization, especially if she finds a new partner. She must understand that her family will now be complete. Ideally, suitable patients for this operation are > 35 years of age.

   - It is a surgical procedure with all the inherent risks of a general anaesthetic. There is a 1:10 000 risk of death from a general anaesthetic.

   - The procedure is usually performed laparoscopically (keyhole surgery) but may need to be converted to a mini-laparotomy and thus leave a bigger surgical scar.

   - The procedure has a 1:200 lifetime risk of failure.

- Early complications include a < 5% risk of bleeding, infection or trauma to the organs and there is a small risk of late complication of an ectopic pregnancy.
- Reversal of the procedure costs £2500 and may not be available on the NHS. The success rate of the reversal operation ranges from 25% to 70% depending on the surgeon and whether a microscope is employed. Alternatively, IVF (*in-vitro* fertilization) treatments are expensive and again not available on the NHS.
- The benefit is that she will be sterilized permanently. It is a single procedure and relatively safe. It is highly effective.

4. **Help** her decide. Ask if she has understood everything or needs clarification.

5. **Explain** the procedure. Through keyhole surgery, i.e. a cut below the umbilicus, her tubes will be permanently clipped with Filschie clips.

6. **Return** for follow-up. She may need time to digest all you have discussed with her. Offer her another appointment if she would like to discuss the consent form with her partner in detail before she signs the form.

Station 10: Answers

1. This is an abnormal ECG.

2. The rate is 70.

3. The rhythm is normal sinus.

4. The axis is normal. The main deflections in leads I and II are positive.

5. The P wave is normal. The P–R interval is normal. The QRS complexes are normal.

6. There are Q waves in leads V1–3 suggestive of an anterior myocardial infarction.

Station 11: Answers

This is a popular PLAB 2 OSCE station! You must know your CPR.

The answers provided are obtained from the *Advanced Life Support Manual* published by the UK Resuscitation Council.

1. **Ensure the safety of rescuer and victim.** Check that it is safe to approach. Look around the park. Ensure that his dog is not loose and about to bite you.

2. **Check the victim and see if he responds.** Approach the manikin, shake his shoulders gently and shout out, 'Hello. Are you all right? Can you hear me?'

3. The manikin is quiet. **Shout for help. Position the manikin gently onto its back.**

4. Place your hand on the manikin's forehead and tilt the head back gently. **Remove any visible obstruction from the manikin's mouth,** including dislodged dentures in an old man. Be seen to be sweeping your finger in the manikin's mouth. **Tilt the chin to open the airway.**

5. Keeping the airway open, put your ear to the manikin's mouth and **listen for breathing for 10 seconds. Look at the chest for movements.** Simultaneously, feel the neck for the carotid pulse. There is none.

6. Look around. If there is no one around, use your mobile phone or search the man's jacket pockets for his mobile and call 999. If you cannot find a mobile phone, then **leave the victim and go for assistance yourself. Make the telephone call and return to the victim.**

    If there is someone nearby, yell out, '**Help! You there. Call 999 and ask for the ambulance service not police!** Tell them this man is not breathing and we are in the middle of Hyde Park. I am wearing a navy blue coat and will jump up and down when I hear the ambulance sirens so they can locate us. Then come back to me and tell me they are on their way.' Otherwise you will be stranded with the victim for hours and will never know if help is on its way.

7. **Give two slow, effective rescue breaths** and make sure you see the chest rise and fall. Ensure head tilt and chin lift. Pinch the vestibule of the nose with the index finger and thumb of your hand on the manikin's forehead. Maintain chin lift as you place your lips around the manikin's mouth ensuring a good seal.

8. **Check for carotid pulse for 10 seconds. If none is present, commence 15 chest compressions** over the middle of the lower half of the sternum and depress the sternum between 4 and 5 cm downwards. Give two breaths in a **ratio of 15:2 compressions and breaths. Every minute, check for signs of circulation but take no more than 10 seconds each time.**

9. Continue until help arrives or you become exhausted.

Station 12: Answers

1. Remark on the view in which the chest X-ray was taken. 'This is a PA view of the chest.'

2. The obvious abnormality is the presence of diffuse alveolar shadowing suggestive of pneumocystis carinii pneumonia. I would suggest that the patient be counselled and offered HIV testing.

3. Remark on the heart, mediastinum, hila, diaphragm, root of the neck and trachea, lung fields, soft tissues, and bones.

Station 13: Answers

1. Examine the patient upright for any apparent varus or valgus deformity and confirm inability to weight-bear.

2. With the patient lying supine, look at the affected knee joint. Look for scars, redness, swelling and/or muscle atrophy of the quadriceps.

3. Note the position of the knee, i.e. whether it is flexed or hyper-extended, lying in the valgus or varus position. Note any limb shortening.

4. Feel the knee for warmth or erythema.

5. Test the knee joint for fluid by cross-fluctuation. This is performed by squeezing the fluid from the suprapatellar pouch downwards with the left hand while the right hand straddles the knee joint below the patella, then repeating this action but keeping the left hand still and squeezing upwards with the right hand positioned below the patella. This should result in fluctuation across the joint if fluid is present.

6. If asked for other tests for fluctuation, mention the patella tap. This is performed by compressing the suprapatellar pouch with the left hand and pushing the patella backwards with the right index finger. The patella tap test is positive if the patella bounces off the femur.

7. Palpate for synovial thickening with the knee in extension. Attempt to lift the patella forward with the thumb and middle finger. If the synovium is thickened, the fingers will not be able to grasp the patella.

8. Palpate for localized tenderness with the knee extended and flexed. In the latter position, the joint line can be easily palpated.

9. Test the knee joint for movement, i.e. flexion, extension, abduction, adduction, lateral and medial rotation. Normal full extension is recorded at 0° and flexion ranges from 0 to 150°. Abduction and adduction are tested with the knee extended. Abduction is movement of the leg with the toes pointed outward, and adduction is movement of the leg with the toes pointed towards the midline. Lateral and medial rotation is tested with the hip and knee flexed 90°.

10. Test the knee joint for stability. The medial and lateral collateral ligaments are tested by holding the right heel of the extended leg with the right hand and supporting the undersurface of the knee with the left hand and then stressing the knee joint in varus and valgus positions. Laxity will be demonstrated if present in either ligament.

    The anterior and posterior cruciate ligaments are tested by the drawer test or the anteroposterior glide. This test involves positioning both knees at 90°. First observe the knee for the sag sign, i.e. has the upper end of the anterior tibia dropped back. This is a sign of posterior cruciate ligament laxity. Then sit lightly on the right foot and grasp the upper end of the tibia with both hands and slowly rock the leg forward and backwards to test for a positive anterior or a positive posterior drawer sign.

    The Lachman's test for joint stability is more difficult to perform and involves positioning the knee in 20° flexion, grasping the femur and tibia in each hand and moving the joint surfaces in opposite directions, backwards and forwards to test for laxity.

11. Finally, examine the patellofemoral joint. Observe the shape, position and palpate for localized tenderness behind the patella. The apprehension test for recurrent patella subluxation or dislocation involves pushing the patella laterally while flexing the knee slightly. Resistance to movement is suggestive.

Station 14: Answers

This is a favourite PLAB 2 OSCE station!

1. Explain to the examiner that you would introduce yourself to the patient. Do not address the manikin.

2. If you are male, explain to the examiner that you would ask the patient if she would prefer a female chaperone be present.

3. Explain to the examiner that you would next explain to the patient that you would like to take a cervical smear.

4. In reality, ask the patient to get undressed from the waist downwards behind the curtain, cover herself with the drape provided and let you know when she is ready to be examined.

5. Check that all the items required are present.

6. Have a glass slide prepared with the patient's name and hospital number pencilled in on the ground glass end of the slide.

7. Position the manikin and adjust the light source.

8. Open a sterilized speculum packet. Don a pair of gloves. Familiarize yourself with how to prepare the Cusco's bivalve metal speculum, i.e. the metal flap needs to be fitted over the screw and the screw needs to be loosely engaged. Warm the speculum under running water.

9. Lubricate a warmed speculum with KY gel. **If no KY gel is available, ask for it. This trick has been used in past PLAB 2 exams and will result in an instant fail if you have overlooked this step!**

10. Explain to the examiner that you would inform the patient that you are about to insert the speculum and that you would instruct her to keep her ankles together and gently drop her knees.

11. Inspect the vulva and comment on its appearance. Spread the labia apart gently with the left hand and gently introduce the warmed and lubricated speculum with the blades closed, parallel to the labia and into the vagina. Insert the speculum

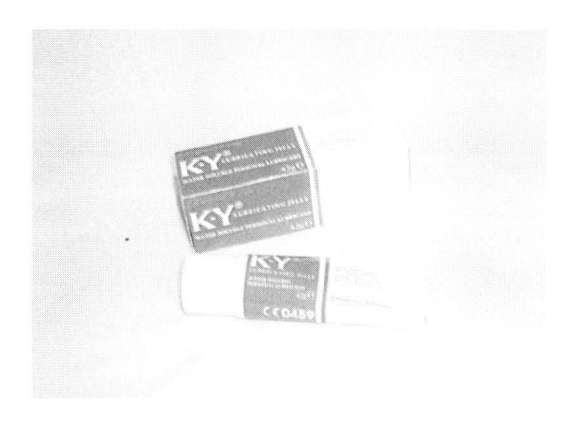

fully, rotate it, open the blades and slowly withdraw until the cervix flops into view. Tighten the screw to secure the position of the speculum with the cervix well demonstrated.

12. Do not clean the cervix before taking a cervical smear. Insert the bilobed end of an Ayre's wooden spatula into the cervical os. Collect cells by rotating the spatula through 360° ensuring that the scrape spans the squamocolumnar junction at all points.

13. Remove the spatula. Loosen the screw, close the blades and gently remove the speculum from the vagina.

14. Spread the material thinly onto the labelled glass slide using gentle longitudinal strokes rather than a circular motion to achieve a single-cell layer.

15. Spray fixative (e.g. Cytofix) generously to the slide.

16. Pour off any excess fixative from the slide after a few minutes.

17. Complete the request form with a ballpoint pen. Place the slide in a slide mailer for dispatch with the request form.

18. Explain to the examiner that you would thank the patient for her cooperation and inform her that the smear will be sent to a laboratory for examination, and that she will be notified of the results by post. She should then have routine cervical smears every 3 years until she is 60 years of age.

Station 15: Answers

This is a favourite PLAB 2 OSCE station!

1. Explain that you would introduce yourself to the patient. Do not address the manikin.

2. Check the patient's identity bracelet.

3. Tell the examiner that you would explain the blood tests to the patient. The blood tests you will carry out are for full blood count to make sure she is not currently anaemic, for sickle cell status if she has not been formally tested, and for a Group and Save specimen to determine her blood group.

4. Check that all your equipment is present. Check the blood tubes. Use a 21-gauge (green needle) and a 20 cc syringe or use a yellow plastic vacutainer and a green or black vacutainer needle.

5. Don a pair of gloves.

6. Apply the tourniquet to the upper arm and proximal to the site of venepuncture. Take care that you do not apply the tourniquet unnecessarily tight.

7. Clean the cubital fossa with an alcohol swab or steret.

8. Select an appropriate vein by gentle palpation.

9. **Advise the patient to look away as you approach** the cephalic, basilic or any other obvious vein with the needle. Warn the patient that she will feel a **sharp scratch**.

10. Approach at an oblique 30–45°. If using the vacutainer, once the vein is pierced, attach each tube to the inside of the vacutainer and the blood will be drawn directly into the tube by suction action. Exchange the tube once full.

11. Once all the necessary blood has been collected, release the tourniquet and cover the area with a piece of cotton gauze as you remove the needle. Ask the patient to bend her arm or raise it up and hold pressure over the site for 3 minutes.

12. **Safe disposal of sharps. You will fail if you do not dispose of sharps appropriately. Do not recap needles** for fear of sharp

injury to yourself. Clear the patient's area. Dispose of all needles in a yellow plastic receptacle labelled SHARPSAFE. Do not overfill the sharps container. On top of the sharps container, there is a particular hole to insert the vacutainer needle for you to unscrew and drop the needle inside. If not, dispose of both the vacutainer needle and holder in the sharps receptacle.

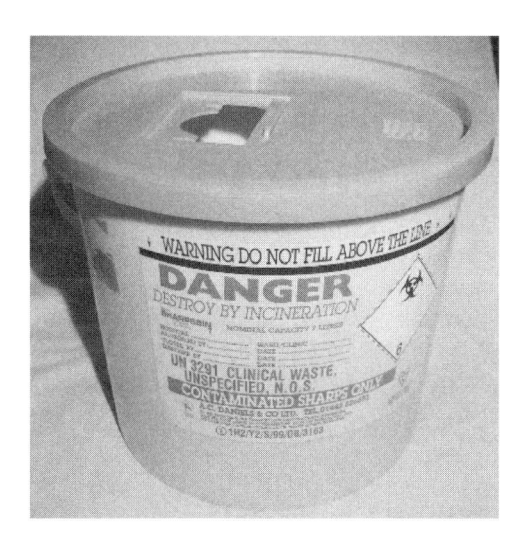

13. Return to the patient. Ask the patient if she is allergic to Elastoplast. If not, place a plaster over the venepuncture site once the bleeding has stopped. If she is allergic, then place a piece of tape over the cotton gauze to secure it.

14. Label the tubes as indicated with the patient's full name, hospital number, date of birth, your name, date and time, and location. A lilac tube top containing citrate is used for full blood count and a purple tube top for the Group and Save specimen. Check that the label on the latter tube reads Group and Save. The latter tube must be hand written. On the request form, request that the Group and Save specimen be frozen, as the operation is more than a week away. Be familiar with the other kinds of blood tubes. Chemistry tests such as U's and E's or urea and electrolytes are collected in the brown tube top, which has no additives. A light blue tube top is used for clotting studies. Glucose is taken in a fluoride-containing tube. Do not rely solely on the colours of the tube tops as these may vary from institution to institution.

15. Place the blood tubes in separate plastic bags and seal the bags. Insert the appropriate blood form with each bag, and thank the patient for her cooperation.

Station 16: Answers

1. This is an abnormal ECG.

2. The rate is 75.

3. The rhythm is normal sinus.

4. The axis is normal. The main deflections in leads I and II are positive.

5. The P waves are normal. The P–R interval should be between 0.12 and 0.22 seconds. The QRS complexes are normal.

6. There is a deep S wave in V2 and a tall R wave in V5. Both add up to greater than seven larger squares suggestive of left ventricular hypertrophy (LVH). LVH can be associated with aortic regurgitation.

7. The ST-waves are inverted in all leads consistent with ischaemia.

Station 17: Answers

1. Explain to the examiner that you would introduce yourself to the patient. Do not address the manikin.

2. Explain to the examiner that you would explain to the patient that the leg wound requires sutures. Explain that it will not hurt, as you will give her a local anaesthetic injection. Explain that she will not require a tetanus booster as her tetanus status is up to date, i.e. last booster within 5 years.

3. Establish that she has full range of movement of the leg and that she has no neurovascular compromise or tendon injury. Have the patient lie in a supine position assuming the wound is on her anterior leg. Don a pair of sterile gloves. Drape the area of the wound with sterile drapes and clean the wound with diluted hydrogen peroxide or betadine using aseptic technique.

4. Prepare a 10-ml syringe with 1–2% lignocaine hydrochloride with adrenaline 1:80,000. The latter is useful to maintain a relatively bloodless field. Warn the patient that she may feel a bee-sting sensation of the local anaesthetic going in. Using a 21-gauge needle attached to the syringe, infiltrate the skin around the wound and the underlying subcutaneous tissues. Always withdraw suction before advancing the needle to ensure that you do not hit a blood vessel.

5. Wait several minutes for the area to be fully anaesthetized. Inform the patient that she will feel pressure but should not feel sharp pain.

6. Close the deeper layer of subcutaneous tissue with inverted absorbable sutures (vicryl or dexon) on a cutting needle. Approximate the skin edges with interrupted non-absorbable nylon or prolene. In the leg, 2–0 suture should be of sufficient strength.

7. Apply steristrips and a sterile gauze dressing over the wound.

8. Explain to the examiner that you would inform the patient that the sutures will need to be removed in a week's time, and that she should make arrangements at her local GP surgery to see the nurse for suture removal.

9. Explain to the examiner that you would inform the patient that if she develops signs of infection, i.e. temperature, wound breakdown, wound discharge, etc., then she should return to Casualty or see her GP for assessment and antibiotics.

10. Explain to the examiner that you would give her painkillers to take home, i.e. paracetamol, ibrufen, coproxamol or co-dydramol, depending on the size and depth of the wound, and that you would thank the patient for her cooperation.

Station 18: Answers

1. Introduce yourself to the patient.

2. Maintain eye contact and avoid medical jargon! Your aim is to reassure the patient.

3. Explain that she has reached menopause and is experiencing symptoms associated with the menopause. Menopause can be confirmed by a blood test for high levels of follicle-stimulating hormone (FSH).

4. Ask her what her understanding is of hormone replacement therapy (HRT) and what if any, are her concerns with taking HRT. This will enable you to reassure her better and dispel any preconceived myths or notions she may already have about HRT.

5. Explain that with the menopause, her levels of oestrogen diminish and that this may be associated with hot flushes, night sweats, palpitations, headaches, vaginal dryness, urinary symptoms and forgetfulness. HRT is given in the form of natural oestrogens and progestogen. Progestogen is given to a woman with a uterus to protect the lining of the womb. The short-term benefits of HRT are as follows: it will improve her short-term memory, increase moisture to the skin, relieve her symptoms of hot flushes and night sweats, give her relief from vaginal dryness and bladder relief from frequent urination as long as a bladder infection has been excluded.

6. Explain that the short-term risks are irregular bleeding and side-effects from progesterone, which may include bloating and weight gain. Reassure her that people react differently and that she may not experience any of these side-effects at all.

7. Explain the long-term benefits of HRT. Inform her that taking HRT is associated with a 2% increase in bone density per year if taken for 5 years, and consequently, it will lessen her risk of osteoporosis by 50%. Inform her that one in two women will suffer a osteoporosis-related fracture in her 70s and that one in four women will suffer a osteoporosis-related fracture in her 60s. Inform her that it has also been associated with a decrease in heart disease by up to 40% and a delay in the onset of Alzheimer's disease.

8. Explain the long-term risks are a twofold increased risk of deep venous thrombosis (DVT) in the first year of use and a 2 per 1000 absolute risk of breast cancer after 5 years of HRT and a 6 per 1000 absolute risk after 10 years of HRT. Reassure her that these risks are very small, and that there is no change in outcome in patients with breast cancer on HRT and those who do not take HRT.

9. Explain that the routes of administration include oral tablets (prempak), transdermal patches, percutaneous, subcutaneous implant, vaginal (vagifem) or as a nasal spray.

10. Checking understanding. Ask the patient if she has any questions or needs further clarification. In fact, it is a good idea to stop frequently and ask, 'Do you understand?'

11. Suggest that she go home and think about what has been discussed to give her time to absorb this.

12. Suggest that she make a follow-up appointment at her convenience if she would like to try HRT.

13. The examiner may ask the actor whether she feels you have put her mind at ease and whether she would like to see you again as a patient.

Station 19: Answers

1. Remark on the view in which the chest X-ray was taken. 'This is a PA view of the chest.'

2. The obvious abnormality is the presence of an encysted pleural effusion in the right base of the lung.

3. Remark on the heart, mediastinum, hila, diaphragm, root of the neck and trachea, lung fields, soft tissues, and bones.

Station 20: Answers

1. This is an abnormal ECG.

2. The rate is 60.

3. The rhythm is normal sinus.

4. There is a left axis deviation. The predominant wave in lead I is the R wave and in lead III is the S wave.

5. The P wave is normal. The P–R interval should be between 0.12 and 0.22 seconds. Each small box represents 0.04 seconds. The QRS complexes are of normal duration.

6. There are diffuse T-wave abnormalities suggestive of ischaemia.

Station 21: Answers

1. The history is suggestive of diabetic ketoacidosis. Treatment includes intravenous cannulation and intravenous fluids, insulin infusion via a pump, insertion of a nasogastric tube as the patient is drowsy and consideration of CVP and Foley urinary catheter insertion for close monitoring of fluid status.

2. Tests to confirm the diagnosis include serum glucose (extreme hyperglycaemia), the presence of 2+ urinary ketones on dipstick, hyperkalaemia, and elevated serum urea and creatinine from dehydration.

3. Take an arterial blood gas. The pH and the HCO_3^- may be reduced.

4. A 0.9% normal saline is the intravenous fluid of choice with 1 litre given over the first 30 minutes followed by 1 l h^{-1} over the next 2 hours. This is then followed by 1 litre over the next 2 hours, 1 litre over the next 3 hours, and so on. Cautious fluid administration should be adopted if there is a co-existent history of heart or renal disease. A central line placement with regular CVP readings is advisable to avoid fluid overload. The patient should have received 6 litres in 11.5 hours. Once the blood glucose is < 10 mmol l^{-1}, switch to 10% dextrose fluid.

5. An insulin regimen involves administration of an intravenous infusion of soluble insulin (Actrapid) 50 units in 50 ml 0.9% saline at 6 units h^{-1} until the blood glucose is < 10 mmol l^{-1}. The insulin infusion can then be halved. Adjust the insulin infusion to maintain the blood glucose between 5 and 10 mmol l^{-1} using insulin in 5–10% dextrose over 8 hours. Continue until the patient can tolerate po. Give the patient preprandial subcutaneous soluble insulin and stop the insulin infusion pump after the meal.

6. Add 40 mmol KCl l^{-1} if the serum K is < 3.5 mmol l^{-1} and withhold if it is > 5 mmol l^{-1}.

7. Replace sodium bicarbonate if pH is 6.9 with aliquots of 200 ml 2.74% HCO_3^- with 15 mmol KCl over 30–60 minutes.

8. Investigate and treat any underlying conditions such as pneumonia, urine infection, etc. Investigations include chest X-ray, blood cultures and midstream urine for culture.

9. Monitoring should include hourly blood glucose, 2 hourly potassium, repeat ABG at 2 hours if the initial ABG was abnormal, continuous ECG monitoring until the potassium level is normal, hourly BP, fluid intake and urine output measurements.

10. Advise the patient that infection may interfere with insulin uptake and that he should not alter his insulin regimen without seeking a medical opinion.

Station 22: Answers

1. This is an abnormal ECG.

2. The rate is 60.

3. The rhythm is normal sinus.

4. There is a left axis deviation. The main deflection in lead I is the positive R wave, and the main deflection in lead III is the negative S wave.

5. The P wave is of normal duration (≤ 0.12 seconds). The P–R interval is normal (between 0.12 and 0.22 seconds) and the QRS complex is normal (≤ 0.10 seconds).

6. There are Q waves in leads V1–4 suggestive of an anteroseptal myocardial infarction.

Station 23: Answers

1. As you will be marked for your written assessment, ensure that you label the right-hand corner of the page with the patient's name and hospital number. Date and time the page in the left-hand column, and write an appropriate heading.

2. Make a heading for **verbal and non-verbal behaviour**. Note the patient's appearance on presentation and behaviour.

3. Comment on his **speech** (rate, retarded or pressure of speech) and content.

4. Make a heading for **mood** – is he suicidal or does he plan to harm others? Is he manic or depressed?

5. Make a heading for **beliefs**. What does he believe about himself or his body? What does he think of others? Does he have any abnormal beliefs (delusions) or ideas of grandiosity or persecution?

6. Make a heading for **unusual experiences or hallucinations**. Note any auditory or visual hallucinations.

7. Make another heading for **orientation**. One form of the Mini Mental State Exam is as follows. Assess cognitive function. Ask him what day of the week it is, day, month, year, the season, where he is, town, building, address and what his name is. Each correct answer is worth one point with a maximum of ten points. Basically, is he oriented to time, place and person?

8. Ask him to take a piece of paper in his right hand, fold it in half with both hands and place it on his lap. Give him one point for each part of the task.

9. Show him a pencil and ask him to identify it. Show him a watch and ask him to identify it. He scores one point for each item correctly identified.

10. Ask him to repeat the sentence you give him: No ifs, ands or buts.

11. Ask him to read what you have written and do what it says. On a sheet of paper, write 'CLOSE YOUR EYES'.

12. Ask the patient to write a complete sentence on a piece of paper. Check for grammar and spelling.

13. Show him a drawing and ask him to copy it, i.e. two intertwined hexagons.

14. **Test his short-term memory.** State three things – apple, chair, penny – and ask him to repeat the three objects. Ask him to remember these three items as you will ask him again in 5 minutes. Ask him to recall those objects in 5 minutes.

15. **Test his concentration.** Ask him to take 7 seconds away from 100, i.e. 93, 86, 79, 72, etc., and give him up to five points.

16. Count the points. The maximum score should be 30. A score of 25–27 is borderline and a score < 25 suggests dementia. Print and sign your name at the end of the written assessment. Note your hospital position and bleep number.

17. **Test his long-term memory.** Ask him who the current monarch is?

Station 24: Answers

1. Introduce yourself to the patient and ask his permission to examine him.

2. **Inspect** the sclera for signs of icterus.

3. Inspect both hands together for tremor, palmar erythema and clubbing.

4. Inspect the chest for gynaecomastia.

5. Inspect the abdomen for scars, striae, spider naevi, visible pulsation, peristalsis, masses, herniae and varicosities. Visible pulsations suggest the abdominal aorta in slim patients or an abdominal aortic aneurysm. Peristalsis from right to left suggest a transverse colon obstruction, and from left to right, a pyloric stenosis. Varicosities or tortuous veins are suggestive of portal vein or inferior vena caval obstruction. If the abdomen is protuberant, think of the five Fs: fat, faeces, flatulence, fluid (ascites) and foetus.

6. Have the patient lying supine on one pillow with his arms by his sides. Ask him to raise his head and cough. Observe for herniae.

7. **Palpation**: ensure you have warmed your hands in front of the examiner. Palpate the four quadrants of his abdomen and look at his face for signs of pain. Initially avoid the area causing the patient pain, in this case the right upper quadrant of the abdomen, until you have completed palpation of the other quadrants. Note any tenderness, rebound or guarding.

8. Gently palpate the right upper quadrant. Palpate the liver 10 cm below the right costal margin and have the patient breath deeply as you palpate upwards 2 cm with each breath. Assess for size, regularity and tenderness. Percuss the liver.

9. Palpate the spleen. Percuss in the mid-axillary line in the tenth interspace.

10. Palpate the kidneys bimanually. Ballott the kidney between your hands.

11. **Percuss** the abdomen for ascites and organ enlargement. To test for shifting dullness, start from the midline and percuss

towards the flanks. If it is dull, reposition the patient on his side and if the uppermost part of the abdomen is now resonant to percussion, this suggests the presence of free intraperitoneal fluid.

12. **Auscultate** for bruits and bowel sounds. Absence of bowel sounds may suggest peritonitis. Increased bowel sounds may suggest obstruction. Succussion splash or splashing may be heard without a stethoscope by moving the abdomen. The presence of a succussion splash suggests a pyloric obstruction.

13. Examine the groin and genitals for herniae and discharge, respectively.

14. Examine the rectum for haemorrhoids, fissures, skin tags and peri-anal warts.

15. Perform a digital rectal examination. At this point, the examiner may ask you to stop. If not, explain that you would use a gloved finger lubricated with KY gel. Ask for KY gel if not present. **You will fail if you do not ask to use this lubricant.** Explain what needs to be done and why to the patient and proceed with the patient turned on his side. If it is a female patient, ask for a female nurse chaperone. Palpate the size of the prostate and its consistency. Palpate for any masses. Check your gloved finger for blood, mucous or pus. Check the stool for blood.

Station 25: Answers

1. This is an abnormal ECG.

2. The rate is 65.

3. The rhythm is normal sinus.

4. There is a right axis deviation.

5. There is a right bundle branch block. There is a dominant R wave in V1 and wide QRS complexes lasting > 0.10 seconds, i.e. greater than three little squares.

Station 26: Answers

1. Introduce yourself to the patient. Establish a rapport.

2. **Ask permission** of the patient to examine her eyes.

3. **Note the external appearance of the eye** for lid asymmetry, proptosis, ptosis, etc.

4. **Note the pupils** for symmetry and response to light and accommodation.

5. **Check extra-ocular movements**. Have the patient follow your pencil with her head in one position.

6. **Check fields:** ask the patient to fixate on your nose, have her cover left eye and tell you when she sees your fingers come into view from the perimeter. Compare her response with your field of vision by covering your right eye. Note any blind spots. Repeat with the opposite eye covered.

7. **Measure her corrected visual acuity,** i.e. with her glasses. Use a Snellen chart: 6/6 is normal vision; 6/12 implies that what she sees at 6 m distance, normal people can see at 12 m distance; 6/60 correlates with the big letter A. Progressively worse visual acuity is then measured by counting fingers, hand movements, perception of light (PL) to no perception of light (NPL). This patient should have reduced vision. The history is extremely suggestive of acute angle closure glaucoma. Angle closure glaucoma is common in elderly women who are far-sighted. Women have smaller anterior chambers and far-sightedness is associated with a smaller sized eyeball. Onset occurs at night when the pupil dilates and consequently closes off the angle.

8. **Note the site of conjunctival injection.** Is it central cornea or peripheral in location? Is it temporal, nasal or medial or lateral canthal?

9. **Assess for relative afferent pupillary defect (RAPD).** Have the patient look in the distance in a darkened room. Shine a light in the right eye and the pupil will constrict. Shine a light in the left eye and the pupil will constrict. Go back to the right eye and if the pupil dilates paradoxically, the patient has an optic nerve injury. This is the Marcus–Gunn test. The patient is then

said to have RAPD in the right eye. In this case, you would expect the patient to have frozen pupils.

10. **Check Ishihara colour vision.** Red is first to be lost, then green in cases of optic neuritis, nerve transection or macular degeneration. Red desaturation can also be measured by using a red pen and asking the patient to score brightness of the red colour out of ten for each eye.

11. **Do not dilate patients with acute angle closure glaucoma!**

12. **At the 30-second bell.** In this patient, a quick feel of the eyeball will confirm a rock hard eye with pressures of 60–80 mmHg. Management for acute angle closure glaucoma includes administration of an anti-emetic and intravenous diamox (acetazolamide) and making an urgent referral to the ophthalmologist on call. The patient has 6–8 hours before losing vision and ending up with PL vision!

Station 27: Answers

1. Remark on the view in which the film was taken. 'This is a PA view of the chest.'

2. 'This patient has diffuse lung shadowing suggestive of aspiration pneumonia.'

3. Remark on the heart, mediastinum, hila, diaphragm, root of the neck and trachea, lung fields, soft tissues, and bones.

Station 28: Answers

1. This ECG shows an electronic pacemaker rhythm with a rate of 70. Electronic pacemakers are fitted for second- or third-degree (complete) AV block. Anticoagulation is mandatory.

2. There is a left axis deviation with the main deflection in lead I being positive, and the main deflection in lead III being negative.

Station 29: Answers

This is a favourite PLAB 2 OSCE station!

1. Introduce yourself to the patient and ask permission to take his blood pressure.

2. Measure the size of his right upper arm. If there is no tape measure available, then hazard a guess. A standard pneumatic cuff is used for arm circumferences between 24 and 32 cm. If the patient is obese, you must ask for a large-sized cuff or reach for one if there is one provided. **You will fail if you use the wrong-sized cuff!**

3. Measure the patient's blood pressure seated initially.

4. Wrap the sphygomomanometer cuff around the upper arm.

5. Inflate the cuff until the pressure exceeds the arterial pressure and the radial pulse is no longer palpable.

6. Place the diaphragm of the stethoscope over the brachial artery just below the cuff.

7. Reduce the cuff pressure slowly until Phase 1 of the Korotkoff sounds is heard. This is the systolic pressure.

8. Deflate the cuff further until the Korotkoff sounds disappear completely. This is Phase 5 or the diastolic pressure. Inflate the cuff and note Phases I and V of the Korotkoff sounds. Phases II–IV describe when the sounds disappear, reappear and become muffled. Do not be misled.

9. A blood pressure of 120/80 is normal, but the normal range can be higher in an elderly individual. Any reading > 150 systolic and 90 diastolic is considered abnormal.

10. Explain that you would also like to take the patient's blood pressure with him standing to exclude postural hypotension. Standing may cause a slight reduction of the systolic pressure of < 20 mmHg and an increase in the diastolic pressure of ≤ 10 mmHg. With postural (orthostatic) hypotension, a large postural fall in blood pressure is associated with dizziness. Take the blood pressure with the patient standing.

11. Thank the patient and note your measurements.

12. **For bonus points,** explain that you would take the patient's blood pressure in the left arm, if you suspected supravalvular aortic stenosis in which the systolic pressure in the right arm is higher than the left.

13. **For bonus points,** explain that you would take the blood pressure in his lower extremities if you suspected aortic coarctation in which the upper extremities are hypertensive and the femoral pulses are weak and delayed.

Station 30: Answers

1. One mental test examination is described below. For this particular test, the maximum score is 34 and normal is ≥ 29. It may be used to obtain serial measurements over time. Each correct answer scores one point unless noted otherwise.

2. Introduce yourself to the patient. Explain that you would like to perform a mental test.

3. Ask the patient for his name and age.

4. Ask for the time to the nearest hour and the time of day.

5. Give the patient a name and a two-line address to repeat in 5 minutes. The maximum score is six with zero to two for each section.

6. Ask for the day of the week, date of the month and current year.

7. Ask for the name of the hospital, ward and town.

8. Ask him if he recognizes two people. This question scores a maximum of two points.

9. Ask him for his birthday, town of birth and the name of a school he has attended.

10. Ask him about his former occupation.

11. Ask for his wife's name.

12. Ask for the name of the Queen and Prime Minister.

13. Ask him to tell you the years for the First and Second World Wars.

14. Ask him to recite the months of the year backwards. This counts for up to two points.

15. Ask him to count to one to 20. This counts for up to two points.

Station 30 Answers

16. Ask him to count backwards from 20 to one. This counts for up to two points.

17. Tally up the score.

Station 31: Answers

This is a favourite PLAB 2 OSCE station!

1. Introduce yourself to the patient.

2. Explain what you are about to do and why.

3. Ask a nurse to sit in as a chaperone if you are a male candidate.

4. Ask the patient to undress from the waist down and close the curtains around her. Give her a sheet to cover her waist.

5. Have her lie down and adjust the light to obtain a good view.

6. Ask her to put her feet together and drop back her knees.

7. Don a pair of gloves and **ask the examiner for KY gel if it is not on display. This is a common tactic to catch you out and will result in an instant fail for this station.** Lubricate your gloved fingers.

8. Examine the vulva and perineum.

9. Gently open the labia majora with one hand and insert your well-lubricated gloved index and middle fingers into the vagina. Assess for adnexal masses and the uterus bimanually. Assess for adnexal tenderness and for cervical motion tenderness (CMT), which is suggestive of pelvic inflammatory disease.

10. Suggest to the examiner that you would proceed to a speculum examination.

Station 32: Answers

1. This is an abnormal ECG.

2. The rate is 135.

3. The rhythm is irregular.

4. There are no P waves. The patient has an irregular rate and irregular rhythm ECG suggestive of atrial fibrillation. This common arrhythmia occurs in 5–10% of the population > 65 years of age. Atrial fibrillation may be the only presenting feature of hyperthyroidism.

Station 33: Answers

Function	Response	Score
Eye opening	spontaneous	4
	to speech	3 (respond to shouting or speech)
	to pain	2 (can be tested by sternal rub or supra-orbital pressure)
	none	1
Best verbal response	orientated	5 (to person, place and time)
	confused conversation	4 (responds, but at times disoriented)
	inappropriate words	3 (random speech)
	incomprehensible sounds	2 (moaning)
	none	1
Best motor response	obeys commands	6
	localizes (response to pain)	5 (can be tested by pressing down on the fingernail bed or by applying supra-orbital or sternal pressure)
	flexes – normal	4 (patient withdraws to pain)
	abnormal	3 (patient responds by decorticate posturing to painful stimuli. The position of the upper limbs is likened to a rabbit with its raised paws)
	extends (to pain)	2 (patient responds by limb extension, i.e. adduction, internal rotation of the shoulder and pronation of the forearm)
	none	1

Note that the minimum score a 'dead' person can receive is three and not zero.

Station 34: Answers

1. This is an abnormal ECG.

2. The rate is 52 bpm.

3. The rhythm is sinus.

4. There is left axis deviation, with the predominant wave in lead I being positive and the predominant wave in lead III being negative.

5. The obvious abnormalities are:
   - First-degree AV block: P–R interval > 0.22 seconds, i.e. greater than five little squares. Normal P–R interval is between 0.12 and 0.22 seconds.
   - Old inferior myocardial infarct with Q waves in leads II, III and aVF.
   - Old anterior infarct with Q waves in leads V1–3. There is also no R wave progression in the anterior leads suggesting damage to the anterior myocardium.

Station 35: Answers

1. Remark on the view in which the film was taken. 'This is a PA and lateral view of the chest.'

2. 'The obvious abnormality is the presence of patchy consolidation suggestive of *Staphylococcus* pneumonia.'

3. Remark on the heart, mediastinum, hila, diaphragm, root of the neck and trachea, lung fields, soft tissues, and bones.

Station 36: Answers

1. Ensure that the ophthalmoscope is working. Turn it on and check the light source.

2. Ideally, ask for a female chaperone when darkening the room if you are a male doctor. There has been an increase in medicolegal cases concerning patients accusing eye doctors of sexual assault in a darkened room!

3. Stand alongside the patient and have him remove his spectacles and fixate on a particular object at the far corner of the room.

4. Remove your spectacles.

5. Dial up the appropriate lens to correct for the refractive error: − lenses correct myopia and + lenses correct hypermetropia.

6. Use your right eye to examine the patient's right eye and your left eye to examine the patient's left eye.

7. First, check the patient's lens for opacities. To do this, dial up to the high + red numbers. In the normal patient, there should be a red reflex until the retina focuses. An absent red reflex suggests opacities or cataracts.

8. When the retina is in focus, examine the optic disc, which should have sharp borders and a central cup. In glaucoma the optic disc may be atropic and grossly cupped.

9. Note any pallor or swelling.

10. Consider dilating the pupil to examine the retina and macula. Make sure that the patient is not driving himself home and that he has a companion to do so. Do not give long-acting mydriatics such as atropine, which has been known to last up to 21 days! It is illegal to drive with a dilated pupil. Use 0.5–1% tropicamide, a short-acting mydriatic that lasts for 3 hours.

11. **Do not dilate a patient with suspected angle closure glaucoma.** In other words, beware of the elderly female who is long-sighted for she is more at risk of developing angle closure glaucoma.

Station 37: Answers

1. Explain to the examiner that you would greet and introduce yourself to the patient. Do not address the manikin.

2. Explain what you are about to do to the examiner.

3. Check that all your equipment is present. Check the identity of the patient (wrist identity bracelet).

4. Make initial preparations. Don a pair of gloves. Open the venflon packet. In resuscitation situations, select the 14- or 16-gauge venflon. Here, a 18-gauge green venflon is adequate.

5. Don a pair of gloves.

6. Apply a tourniquet to the upper arm.

7. Select a vein by gentle palpation over the cubital fossa.

8. Cleanse the area over the selected vein with an alcohol steret.

9. Palpate the vein with your left fingers and slowly advance the cannula into the vein. Approach the vein at an oblique angle. As soon as you see blood return or flashback, advance the plastic sheath while withdrawing the introducer.

10. Release the tourniquet.

11. Open a packet of gauze. Place some dressing gauze under the venflon to absorb any blood spillage as you compress the proximal end of the cannulated vein with your left fingers and withdraw the needle with your right hand. Cap the venflon.

12. Place a clear adhesive, i.e. vecafix, over the venflon to secure it in place.

13. Fill a 10-ml syringe with normal saline from the 10-ml ampoule provided and flush the cannula.

14. Explain to the examiner that you would thank the patient for her cooperation. You will also be marked on how fluently and professionally you have performed the procedure.

Station 38: Answers

1. Politely introduce yourself to the patient.

2. Ask the patient to lie flat and straight on the couch.

3. Ask the patient to point out the site of the pain and where it radiates.

4. Inspect the legs for shortening or rotation, scars, sinuses, muscle bulk or wasting.

5. Bilaterally palpate the hip joint to compare the distance between the anterior superior iliac spine and the top of the trochanter.

6. Turn the patient on his side and imagine a line from the anterior superior iliac spine to the ischial tuberosity – Nelaton's line. If the top of the greater trochanter is above this line, there is shortening of the femur or a dislocation of the hip.

7. Is there any limb shortening – real or apparent? Use a tape measure to confirm.

8. Check movement. Do a Thomas's test for fixed flexion. Place your left hand underneath the patient's backside. Grasp one leg and flex the hip and knee until you feel the spine press against your hand. If the other hip joint is normal, that thigh will remain flat on the couch, i.e. no fixed flexion. If there is fixed flexion deformity, the thigh will lift up from the couch. Repeat on the opposite side.

9. Check for passive movements of flexion, extension, abduction, adduction and internal and external rotation. When testing flexion, place your fingers on the greater trochanter and your thumb on the iliac spine so that you can detect any pelvic tilting. When testing abduction and adduction, keep your fingers and thumb stretched across the iliac spines to detect any movement of the pelvis. When testing rotation, flex the hip and the knee to 90° and rotate the femur by moving the foot back and forth across the line of the limb.

10. Check for active movements and range of movements against resistance (power).

11. Ask the patient to stand up. Check for stability.

12. Perform the Trendelenburg test. Ask the patient to stand on one leg. The opposite side of the pelvis should rise. If the opposite buttock falls, the test is positive. Implications of a positive Trendelenburg include paralysed adductor muscles, an unstable joint (fracture of the neck of the femur or a congenital dislocation of the hip) or approximation of the insertion and origin of the abductor muscles preventing their proper function by a severe coxa vara or a dislocation of the hip.

13. Ask the patient to walk. Examine his poise and gait.

Station 39: Answers

1. Politely greet the patient.

2. Discuss the presenting complaint. Establish the duration of each attack and his dizziness.

3. Ask him to describe what he means by dizziness. Is the room spinning or is he unsteady on his feet? Vertigo versus light-headedness. The patient will acknowledge the former.

4. Ascertain the character of the vertigo. Is the onset acute or insidious, continuous or intermittent? What are the relieving factors and the exacerbating factors?

5. Establish whether there are any associated auditory problems. Has he suffered any hearing loss or tinnitus? He will deny this.

6. Establish whether there are any associated neurological symptoms such as diplopia, dysarthria, hemiplegia, dysphasia, hemiparesis, facial palsy or ataxia. Remember to use layman's terms. He admits to associated ataxia.

7. Establish whether there are any other associated symptoms such as nausea and vomiting, visual loss or amaurosis fugax? He admits to nausea and vomiting made worse when he moves his head.

8. Ask him about his prior medical history – a history of hypertension for how long, cerebrovascular accident, ischaemic heart disease, myocardial infarction, etc.

9. Ask him about his drug history.

10. At the 30-second bell, suggest vertebrobasilar transient ischaemic attacks (TIAs). Classically vertebrobasilar TIAs are associated with transient episodes of vertigo and ataxia, nystagmus, visual loss and/or dysarthria. Carotid TIAs are associated with a hemiplegic stroke or a transient episode of hemiparesis, dysphasia, facial palsy or ipsilateral amaurosis fugax (often described as a blind coming down before their eyes).

Station 40: Answers

1. Remark on the view in which the film was taken. 'This is a PA view of the chest.'

2. 'The obvious abnormality is a mass in the left apex with rib destruction and consolidation. This suggests Pancoast tumour with consolidation.'

3. Remark on the heart, mediastinum, hila, diaphragm, root of the neck and trachea, lung fields, soft tissues, and bones.

Station 41: Answers

1. Politely greet the patient (actor). Establish a rapport.

2. Determine the severity and duration of the present illness.

3. Establish the symptom progression. Establish the alleviating and exacerbating factors for wheezing and dyspnoea.

4. Determine if there are any associated symptoms: coughing, sputum, haemoptysis, orthopnoea, watery rhinorrhoea, nasal blockage, itchy eyes, fever, chest pain, fatigue, etc. She only admits to coughing and orthopnoea.

5. Establish disturbance of sleeping pattern from coughing and wheezing.

6. Exclude possible causative or trigger factors such as to exposure to pets, dust mites, pollen or smoking. She denies all.

7. Ask whether there is a family history or if she has a history of atropy or asthma.

8. She states that her mother suffers from hayfever and asthma.

9. At the 30-second bell, suggest that the most likely diagnosis is new onset asthma.

Station 42: Answers

The duties of a doctor registered with the General Medical Council published by the GMC are as follows:

'Patients must be able to trust doctors with their lives and well being. To justify that trust, we as a profession have a duty to maintain a good standard of practice and care and to show respect for human life. In particular as a doctor you must:

1. make the care of your patient your first concern;

2. treat every patient politely and considerately;

3. respect patients' dignity and privacy;

4. listen to patients and respect their views;

5. give patients information in a way they can understand;

6. respect the right of patients to be fully involved in decisions about their care;

7. keep your professional knowledge and skills up to date;

8. recognize the limits of your professional competence;

9. be honest and trustworthy;

10. respect and protect confidential information;

11. make sure that your personal beliefs do not prejudice your patients' care;

12. act quickly to protect patients from risk if you have good reason to believe that you or a colleague may not be fit to practice;

13. avoid abusing your position as a doctor; and

14. work with colleagues in the ways that best serve your patients' interests.

In all these matters, you must never discriminate unfairly against your patients or colleagues. And you must always be prepared to justify your actions to them.'

Station 43: Answers

1. Introduce yourself to the patient and establish a rapport.

2. Ask permission to perform a breast examination. Ask if she would like a female chaperone to attend.

3. Ask the patient to get undressed from the waist up. Draw the curtain around the patient for privacy. Ask her to call when she is ready to be examined.

4. Ask her to sit facing you on the couch and point to the location of the breast lump.

5. Note the contours and symmetry of her breasts as she sits with her arms by her side, on her hips and raised above her head. Is there any asymmetry, nipple retraction, tethering or obvious masses?

6. Ask the patient to lie down and place her right hand behind her head. Ask her to point again to where she feels the lump. Rub your hands together to warm your palms and gently palpate the right breast. The two techniques commonly used are palpation in a radial pattern in circles from outwards in or following spokes of a wheel.

7. If you palpate a mass, determine whether it is attached to the skin or the pectoral muscles. Have the patient place her hand on her hip to contract the pectoral muscles. Does the lump move? If not, it is attached to the muscle. Note the size, shape, site and consistency of the lump.

8. Check for nipple discharge. Ask the patient to reproduce the discharge. Note any nipple retraction.

9. Palpate the axillary region supporting the patient's arm as you do so.

10. Repeat the breast exam on the left side.

11. In the patient's case, a cystic lump is palpated. You are obliged to perform a fine-needle aspiration biopsy (FNAB) and send it off for cytology. You may be asked how to perform a FNAB.

Station 44: Answers

This is a favourite PLAB 2 OSCE station!

1. Introduce yourself to the patient and establish a rapport.

2. Ask her to join you in a private room. Offer her a chair.

3. Speak slowly and softly. Explain that despite all efforts to help Mr Barton's breathing, he has passed away. Offer her a box of tissues if she becomes tearful.

4. Put a hand on her shoulder, back or over her hand to offer support.

5. Express your deepest sympathy and sorrow for what has happened.

6. Ask her if she has any questions about what has happened and what will happen now.

7. Explain that as the cause of her husband's sudden death is unclear, the coroner will be requesting a post mortem. Explain that this requires consent to be given by her.

8. Ask her whether she understands what is meant by a post mortem.

9. Explain that a post mortem is an examination of the deceased and his organs to determine the cause of his death. Explain that this information is confidential.

10. Explain that there are four types of post mortems. A full post mortem is offered to verify the cause of death and to study the reasons why. A small sample of each organ will be sent for examination. The brain, however, will need to be put in a solution for at least 5 days to allow detailed examination and is then returned to the body. For some brain abnormalities, this may need to be longer and the funeral may be delayed. This type of full post mortem includes removal of small fragments of tissue for medical education and research.

11. Explain that a second type of post mortem is a full post mortem with the omission of removal of tissue for medical education and research.

12. Explain that a third type of post mortem is a limited post mortem to examine specified organs and involves a surgical incision.

13. Explain that a fourth type of post mortem involves needle biopsies of organs and does not involve a surgical incision. It is an external examination, which includes X-rays and medical photographs.

14. Explain that the body is returned intact and in a timely fashion for burial to be arranged with the funeral director at her family's convenience.

15. Explain that a post mortem will ultimately help her and her family to understand why this has happened and eventually help obtain closure in the grieving process.

16. Explain that a post mortem may expedite insurance claims as a clear cause of death can be established.

17. Ask her if she has any questions. Give her time to read the consent form for a post mortem before she signs and dates below.

18. Ask her if she recalls whether he has consented to organ donation or possesses an organ donation card at home.

19. Ask her if she would like to spend some time alone with her deceased husband and offer to help her contact family members.

Station 45: Answers

1. Introduce yourself to the patient and establish a rapport.

2. Note the appearance of the patient and how she interacts with you. What is her effect like? Does she avoid eye contact?

3. Start with an open-ended question and ask her about her childhood and adolescence. This will help her relax and express herself in her own words.

4. Gear the conversation towards the present complaint. How long has the weight loss and depression been bothering her? Did any life event trigger this problem?

5. What was her premorbid condition like? Was she always depressed or is this a recent change?

6. What is the patient's insight into her own problem? How would she like you to help her?

7. Ask specific questions about her weight loss. How much weight has she lost and over what period? Does she binge eat or induce vomiting?

8. Ask specific questions about her amenorrhoea. When did her periods stop? Had her menstrual cycles been regular? Does she exercise excessively?

9. Ask specific questions about her depression. Is her sleep pattern disturbed? Does she have trouble going to sleep? Does she wake up early? Conversely, does she sleep too much? Has she lost her appetite? Does she feel tired all the time? How does she see her future? Has she ever considered harming herself or thought about suicide?

10. Ask about any personal or family history of psychiatric illness.

11. Ask her about her social habits. Does she drink alcohol, smoke or indulge in recreational drugs?

12. At the 30-second bell, suggest that she may be suffering from anorexia nervosa and depression. Suggest that you would like to perform a physical examination for evidence of anorexia

such as ketone breath, lanugo hair, acid burns in the oral cavity, etc. and would arrange for blood tests to exclude metabolic disorders. Suggest psychotherapy and SSRI (anti-depressants) if the diagnosis is confirmed.

Station 46: Answers

1. Introduce yourself to the patient and establish a rapport.

2. Ask permission of the patient to examine his shoulders.

3. Ask the patient to remove his shirt.

4. Ask the patient to point to where it hurts and to where the pain radiates.

5. Look at the affected shoulder joint. Is there any winging of the scapula, wasting of the deltoid or supraspinatus muscle, joint swelling or any other deformity? What position is the patient holding his arm.

6. Compare both shoulders from the front and back of the patient.

7. Palpate the affected shoulder joint. Is the skin warm, i.e. is the joint inflamed? Palpate for any joint effusions. Palpation should begin at the sternoclavicular joint, along the clavicle to the acromoclavicular joint, and proceed to the anterior edge of the acromion and around the acromion to the back of the joint. Note any tenderness or crepitus.

8. Test active movements of the shoulder joint. Observe the patient from the front and then from behind. Check for abduction from 0° (arms by his side) to 180° (arms up above the head and hands together). Abduction is initially achieved at the glenohumeral joint by the supraspinatus muscle and is then taken over by the scapula. The last 60° of abduction is scapulothoracic and uses the deltoid muscle. Consequently, pain initially is more likely due to rotator cuff tear or supraspinatus tendinitis and pain at the end of abduction is more likely due to acromioclavicular arthritis.

9. Flexion and extension are tested by asking the patient to raise his arms forwards and upwards and then down and behind. Flexion uses the pectoralis major, deltoid and coracobrachialis muscles. Extension uses the deltoid muscle. If the shoulder is initially flexed, the muscles of extension are the latissimus dorsi, pectoralis major and teres major.

10. Adduction is tested by asking the patient to move his arms across the front of his body and uses the pectoralis major, latissimus dorsi, teres major and subscapularis muscles.

11. External and internal rotation are tested by asking the patient initially to flex his elbows at 90° and to hold his arms against the sides. External rotation is achieved by moving the hands outwards (normal is 80°) and internal rotation is achieved by bringing in his hands across the body or by pacing the back of the hand against the lumbar spine and moving the elbows forward. The patient is then asked to clasp his fingers behind his neck (external rotation in abduction). Finally, the patient is asked to reach up his back with his fingers from both hands (internal rotation in adduction).

12. Stabilizing the scapula tests passive movements. Place your hand firmly on top of the patient's shoulder to keep the scapula anchored.

13. Movement of the scapula on the chest wall is tested by asking the patient to shrug his shoulders (elevation), depress his shoulders, punch (forward action) and brace his shoulders (retraction).

14. Power:
    - Deltoid: the patient abducts against resistance.
    - Serratus anterior (long thoracic nerve C5–7): the patient is asked to push against a wall with both hands.
    - Pectoralis major: the patient is asked to thrust both hands onto his hips.
    - Trapezius: the patient is asked to shrug his shoulders against resistance.

15. Thank the patient at the end of the examination.

Station 47: Answers

1. Introduce yourself to the patient and establish a rapport.

2. Ask permission to examine her hands.

3. Ask her which is her dominant hand.

4. Compare both hands. Look for scars, wasting, colour, hair, lumps or deformities.

5. Look at the nails for pitting (psoriasis), koilonychia, etc.

6. Feel the temperature and texture of the skin. Note the pulse.

7. Test active movements. Asking the patient to curl her fingers up with her palms facing upwards tests flexion. Ask the patient to touch the tip of each of her fingers with the tip of her thumb.

8. Test for passive movements in a similar fashion.

9. Test the patient's grip strength by having her squeeze your fingers.

10. Conduct a neurological assessment to ascertain the distribution of the tingling and numbness. The median nerve supplies sensation to the palmar aspect of the radial three and a half fingers, the dorsal aspect of the distal phalanx and half of the middle phalanx of the same fingers. The ulnar nerve supplies sensation to the ulnar one and a half fingers and the skin over the hypothenar eminence. The radial nerve supplies sensation to the lateral aspect of the first metacarpal and the back of the first web space. Test for light touch, two-point discrimination and pinprick.

11. Nerve palsies: a median nerve palsy causes wasting of the thenar eminence, absent flexion of the distal interphalangeal joint of the index finger, absent abduction and opposition of the thumb. An ulnar nerve palsy causes wasting of the hypothenar eminence and hollows between the metacarpals, absence of flexion of the ring and little fingers and absence of adduction and abduction of the fingers. A radial nerve palsy causes absence of wrist extension and extension of the metacarpophalangeal joints and of the thumb interphalangeal joint.

12. A quick test for the median nerve is to have the patient abduct the thumb (raise the thumb to the ceiling) with his palm facing upwards. To test the radial nerve, ask the patient to extend his wrist from a flexed position. To test the ulnar nerve, ask the patient to separate his little finger from the rest of his fingers in a sideways manner (abduction).

13. Specific tests. Test for Tinel's sign. Tap on the palmar aspect of the wrist of the affected hand over the flexor retinaculum sheath. This should elicit symptoms of tingling in the fingers in the distribution of the median nerve which lies beneath the sheath. This is a positive Tinel's sign.

14. Test for Phalen's sign. Ask the patient to flex both wrists and press the back of both her hands together with the fingers pointing to the floor. This should also recreate her symptoms by putting pressure on the flexor retinaculum, which in turn compresses the median nerve.

15. Pearl of wisdom: Froment's sign. This is not a test for carpal tunnel syndrome but is a favourite examination question when it comes to the hand. Test for Froment's sign. Ask the patient to grip a piece of paper between her thumbs and index fingers and attempt to pull it away. If the patient flexes her thumb, she has a weak adductor pollicis and the flexor pollicis longus is compensating.

16. Pearl of wisdom. Know how to test whether the vascular supply to the hand is obtained from both the radial and the ulnar arteries or solely by the radial artery. This is important to know when performing radial artery cannulation. The test is performed as follows. Ask the patient to squeeze his hand shut tightly. Compress the patient's radial artery firmly with the tips of your index and middle fingers. Ask the patient to open his hand slowly. Do not release pressure on the patient's radial artery. If the hand turns pink, the ulnar artery also supplies it. If the hand remains white, the hand relies solely on the radial artery for its circulation.

17. At the 30-second bell, suggest a diagnosis of carpal tunnel's syndrome.

Station 48: Answers

1. Introduce yourself to the patient and establish a rapport.

2. Ask the patient when the symptoms began. Do they correlate with starting the oral contraceptive pill?

3. Ask her to describe the headache. Where does it start and radiate? Is the pain sharp, throbbing or dull in nature? What are some trigger factors? Are they stress, premenstrual tension, chocolate overindulgence (high in phenylethylamine), red wine or cheese (high in tyramine)? Does anything relieve the headache? Does a darkened room help?

4. Ask her about any associated symptoms. Your aim is to exclude other causes of headaches such as tension, meningitis, subarachnoid haemorrhage, space-occupying lesion, etc. Does she see flashes of light, an aura preceding the headache (migraine)? Does she suffer from neck pain or stiffness and drowsiness (meningism)? Is the pain unilateral and behind the eye and worse at night (cluster headache)? Has she suffered any recent head trauma? Is the headache the worst headache she has ever experienced (subarachnoid haemorrhage)? Does the headache feel like a tight band constricting her head or does she have pain at the back of her head (tension)?

5. Ask about any family history of migraines or bleeds in the brain?

6. Ask the patient if she has anything further to add or has any questions.

7. At the 30-second bell, suggest a diagnosis of migraine. Suggest first-line treatment with paramax (500 mg paracetamol and 5 mg metoclopramide), two tablets every 4 hours prn.

Station 49: Answers

1. Explain to the examiner that you would introduce yourself to the patient. Do not address the manikin.

2. Explain to the examiner that you would explain to the patient that you would like to administer an anti-emetic intravenously (in layman's terms).

3. Check that you have all the necessary equipment: needle, syringe, alcohol steret wipe, gloves, ondansetron vial and normal saline flush.

4. Check the patient's drug chart, the patient's identity bracelet, and the dose and date of expiry on the ondansetron vial. Request that a second person read the vial with you to verify the dose and date of expiry on the glass vial.

5. Explain to the examiner that you would check with the patient that she has no known drug allergies.

6. Don a pair of gloves.

7. Attach a needle to a syringe.

8. Break the glass vial along the line indicated.

9. Draw up 8 mg into the syringe. Check how many milligrams are in each millilitre.

10. Clean the cannula portal with an alcohol steret wipe.

11. Inject 8 mg ondansetron slowly into the cannula.

12. Prepare a normal saline flush in a drawn-up syringe.

13. Flush the cannula with 5–10 ml normal saline.

14. Close the cannula portal.

15. Dispose of all sharps in the appropriate receptacle. **Do not recap any needles.** Tidy up after yourself.

16. Explain to the examiner that you would thank the patient for her cooperation.

Station 50: Answers

1. Remark on the view that the film was taken. 'This is a PA view of the chest.'

2. 'The obvious abnormality is right paratracheal lymphadenopathy suggestive of tuberculosis.'

3. Remark on the heart, mediastinum, hila, diaphragm, root of the neck and trachea, lung fields, soft tissues, and bones.

Station 51: Answers

1. Explain to the examiner that you would introduce yourself to the patient. Do not address the manikin.

2. Explain to the examiner that you would tell the patient that she has had an anaphylactic (allergic) response to eating nuts and that it is necessary for you to administer adrenaline intramuscularly. Explain that this is an injection into the muscle of her upper arm (deltoid).

3. Check that you have all the necessary equipment: needle, syringe, alcohol steret wipe, a pair of gloves, vial of adrenaline (1 in 1000), a cotton ball and a plaster.

4. Check the patient's drug chart, the patient's identity bracelet, and the dose and date of expiry on the vial of adrenaline. Request that a second person read the vial with you to verify the dose and date of expiry details are accurate.

5. Check that the patient has no known drug allergies.

6. Don a pair of gloves.

7. Attach a needle to a 1- or 2-ml size syringe.

8. Break the glass vial along the line indicated.

9. Draw up 0.5 ml (0.5 mg) adrenaline 1 in 1000 into your syringe.

10. Clean the skin on the upper arm over the deltoid muscle with an alcohol steret wipe.

11. Inject 0.5 ml adrenaline into the deltoid muscle. Be careful to avoid the medial and anterior branches of the axillary nerve. The medial branch innervates the posterior part of the deltoid and a small patch of skin over the muscle and the anterior branch curls around the surgical neck of the humerus to innervate the anterior two-thirds of the deltoid. The landmark for this branch is 5 cm below the tip of the acromion.

12. Withdraw the syringe and apply a cotton ball to the site. Ask the patient to apply pressure as you safely dispose of the needle and syringe into a sharps' receptacle. In this case, just tape the cotton ball in place.

13. Normally, you would ask the patient if she is allergic to Elastoplast. If not, remove the cotton ball and apply a plaster. If she is, then place a piece of tape over the cotton ball.

14. If asked to administer an intramuscular injection to the gluteal muscles, beware of the sciatic nerve. The surface landmarks for the nerve are from the midpoint between the ischial tuberosity and greater trochanter to the apex of the popliteal fossa.

15. Explain to the examiner that you would thank the patient for her cooperation.

Station 52: Answers

1. Introduce yourself to the patient and establish a rapport.

2. Ask the patient to tell you more about the palpitations. For how long has he had them and for how long do they last?

3. Ask him to describe the character of the palpitations. Is it rapid and/or irregular? What makes it worse or better? When does it come on? After exercise or at rest?

4. Ask him about any associated symptoms of shortness of breath: exertional, nausea, sweating, dizziness, blackouts, etc? Is the chest tightness similar to his angina? Does he get short of breath at night? How many pillows does he need to sleep with at night?

5. Ask him about his risk factors for cardiac disease. Does he drink alcohol in excess? How many cigarettes or cigars does he smoke each day? Has he suffered from a stroke? Does he have a history of hypertension, ischaemic heart disease (myocardial infarction, MI), hypercholesterolaemia, peripheral vascular disease (intermittent claudication), cerebrovascular accident or diabetes mellitus? Does he have a history of rheumatic fever?

6. Does he have any family history of ischaemic heart disease or hypercholesterolaemia?

7. What are his current medications? Does he have any known drug allergies?

8. At the 30-second bell, suggest that you would like to perform a cardiovascular exam and obtain a 12-lead electrocardiogram next. Suggest that the most likely diagnosis for the patient's rapid and irregular palpitations would be atrial fibrillation or a ventricular tachyarrhythmia.

Station 53: Answers

1. Introduce yourself to the patient and establish a rapport.

2. Ask permission to conduct an examination of her heart and circulation.

3. Inspect the patient. Is she in pain or distress? Does she have a Turner's (co-arctation of the aorta)? Is she of short stature with a webbed neck? Does she have a Down's syndrome body habitus? Is she of short stature with a flat facies, epicanthal folds, slanting eyes and signs of mental retardation? If so, then think she is at risk for ASD or VSD. Does she have Marfan's syndrome (aortic incompetence) with features of arachnodactyly (spider fingers), arm span longer than the height, etc?

4. Examine the patient's face. Inspect the eyes for signs of hyperlipidaemia such as xanthelasma (fatty yellow deposits in the eyelids) or corneal arcus (a white ring around the outer iris). Exclude signs of Grave's disease (lid lag, proptosis, lid retraction). A malar flush may be associated with mitral incompetence. Inspect the fundi for hypertensive changes. Inspect for Argyll–Robertson pupils, which may be seen with syphilitic aortic incompetence. Inspect the eyes for lens dislocation and the mouth for a high arched palate (Marfan's syndrome). Inspect the mucosa for petechiae (infective endocarditis). Inspect the tongues and lips for cyanosis.

5. Examine the patient's hands. Look for signs for infective endocarditis such as splinter haemorrhages (fine, longitudinal haemorrhagic streaks), Osler's nodes (tender nodules on the tips of her fingertips), Janeway lesions (red macules on the wrist and dorsum of the hand). Note any nail-fold infarcts, nicotine stains, clubbing, or tendon xanthomas.

6. Examine the pulse at the radial, carotid and brachial arteries. Note the rate, rhythm, character, and volume. Check the peripheral pulses. Note any radiofemoral delay (co-arctation of the aorta).

7. Take the blood pressure.

8. Examine the jugular venous pulse at the right internal jugular vein. Observe the patient at 45° with the head slightly turned to the left. Observe the internal jugular vein as it passes medial

to the clavicular head of the sternomastoid muscle, behind the angle of the jaw to the ear lobe. It is raised if it is above 3 cm. There are two waveforms: the a wave (atrial contraction) and v wave (end of ventricular systole which represents the maximum venous filling of the right atrium). If the patient has a raised JVP with no pulsations, think superior vena cava obstruction. If the patient has an absent a wave, think atrial fibrillation. If the patient has cannon a waves, think complete heart block, atrial flutter or ventricular tachycardia. This list is not exhaustive. If the patient has a large a wave, think pulmonary hypertension, pulmonary stenosis or tricuspid stenosis. If the patient has systolic (cv) waves, think tricuspid regurgitation. If the patient has a slow y descent, think tricuspid stenosis.

9. Inspect the precordium. Are there any scars from previous operations (lateral thoracotomy or midline sternotomy)? Does she have a pacemaker box?

10. Palpate for the apex beat in the fifth intercostal space in the mid-clavicular line. If it is shifted laterally, think cardiomegaly or mediastinal shift. Assess the character.

11. Auscultate with the bell and the diaphragm at the apex. Listen for the first and second heart sounds and then for any added heart sounds and murmurs. Listen again at the lower left sternal edge, the aortic and the pulmonary areas (right and left of the manubrium). Reposition the patient in the left lateral position and again palpate for the apex beat. Listen for the diastolic rumble of mitral stenosis.

12. Sit the patient up and listen at the lower left sternal border for aortic regurgitation (diastolic murmur accentuated at the end of expiration).

13. Examine the chest. Percuss the back to exclude a pleural effusion and auscultate for inspiratory crepitations of left heart failure.

14. Examine the abdomen. Palpate for hepatomegaly (right ventricular failure) and pulsatility (tricuspid incompetence). Palpate for splenomegaly (endocarditis) and for an abdominal aortic aneurysm. Palpate the femoral arteries and check for bruits.

15. Examine the peripheral extremities for pulses and signs of peripheral vascular disease, oedema, varicose veins, etc. Check

the patient for scars from previous operations. It is important to know in this particular woman whether she has had varicose vein stripping in the past and consequently has no available saphenous veins for grafting.

16. You will not be able to perform a full cardiovascular examination in 5 minutes. Hopefully the examiner will direct you to a particular part of the exam or ask you to omit steps as you go along to expedite the examination. Explain what you are looking for and note any positive findings as you examine the patient.

17. You will also be marked on how fluent and professional you conduct yourself and the examination.

Station 54: Answers

1. Introduce yourself to the patient and establish a rapport.

2. Explain that it is necessary for her to undergo an operation to remove her inflamed or diseased appendix called an appendicectomy. At age 16, she is of legal age to give consent.

3. Ask her what her understanding is of the procedure and what her concerns are.

4. Explain the procedure in layman's terms. Explain that the operation is performed under general anaesthesia. Explain that a small incision will be made on the lower right-hand side of her abdomen and that the abdomen will be opened to identify the appendix. The appendiceal artery, the appendiceal mesentery and the base of the appendix will be clamped, divided and ligated. The appendix will be removed and the appendix stump ligated and buried in a purse-string suture. The peritoneum and muscle layers are closed with absorbable sutures and the skin is closed with interrupted nylon sutures or subcuticular prolene. The skin sutures will need to be removed in a week's time.

5. Explain that the risk of complications is small but needs to be addressed. The possible complications that can arise from this procedure are wound infection, pelvic or abdominal abscess formation, and paralytic ileus. If she developed a wound infection, she would be treated with intravenous antibiotics. If she developed a pelvic abscess that did not respond to antibiotics, she may need a second operation. If she developed a paralytic ileus, she would be managed with intravenous fluids and a nasogastric tube until the ileus settled and her bowels returned to normal function.

6. Explain that the benefits of this operation far outweigh the risks. Explain that an inflamed and infected appendix could rupture and lead to peritonitis and gangrene in the abdominal cavity. This can then lead to death if untreated.

7. Explain that she would be likely to remain in hospital for 3–5 days depending on the speed of her recovery.

8. Ask her if she has understood or whether she needs you to clarify any points.

9. Ask her if she would like to contact any family members and involve them in her decision-making process if she feels unsure.

10. Complete the consent form with the name of the operation and a short list of the complications that can arise. Print, sign and date the consent form.

11. Have her read the consent form, and print, sign and date the form at the bottom.

Station 55: Answers

1. Explain that you would introduce yourself to the patient. Do not address the manikin. You are told that the patient has now lost consciousness.

2. Gently shake the patient's shoulders and ask loudly, 'Are you all right?'

3. Shout for assistance in Casualty.

4. Control his airway. Use a head-tilt with anterior displacement of the mandible (chin-lift and, if necessary, jaw-thrust). Place your hand on his forehead and tilt the head back gently. Remove any visible obstruction from the patient's mouth, including loose dentures. With your fingertips under the point of the patient's chin, lift the chin to open the airway. These manoeuvres will prevent posterior displacement of the tongue and occlusion of the airway.

5. Look for chest movements. Listen at the patient's mouth for breath sounds. Feel for air on your cheek. Do not take more than 10 seconds.

6. If he is not breathing, give two effective breaths. Check if circulation is present by checking the carotid pulse for no more than 10 seconds. It is present in the patient. Proceed to supplemental oxygen therapy.

7. Clear the mouth and pharynx of any secretions gently using a rigid pharyngeal suction tip (Yankauer). Possible complications that may arise from vigorous suctioning and stimulation of the catheter in the mucosa are sudden onset of hypoxaemia, increased arterial pressure and tachycardia, vagal response with bradycardia and hypotension, cardiac arrhythmias, and mucosal injury.

8. Insert an oropharyngeal airway (Guedel size 3–5) based on the distance (in millimetres) from the flange to the distal tip and the size of the adult. Insert the airway backwards as it enters the mouth and rotate the airway as it approaches the posterior wall of the pharynx.

9. Administer oxygen via a Venturi mask. This provides high gas flow with a fixed oxygen concentration. This type of oxygen

delivery is advocated for patients with chronic hypercarbia (COAD) for the treatment of moderate to severe hypoxaemia. Beware the administration of high oxygen concentrations in these patients as a sudden increase in PaO_2 blocks the stimulant effect of hypoxaemia on the respiratory centres. Use the mask with 24% oxygen concentration initially. The patient can then be monitored for respiratory depression, and the concentration of oxygen can then be titrated against PaO_2. If this patient did not have a history of COAD, a face mask with a constant flow of oxygen into the reservoir at 10 l min^{-1} would produce an oxygen concentration of 100%, which is ideal in a cardiac arrest situation.

10. Auscultate the lungs for clear breath sounds during ventilation.

Station 56: Answers

This is a favourite PLAB 2 OSCE station!

1. Explain to the examiner that you would introduce yourself to the patient. Do not address the manikin.

2. Explain to the examiner that you would tell the patient that you would like to perform a rectal examination.

3. In reality, you would now ask the patient to get undressed from the waist down and lie on the examining couch.

4. Position the manikin on its left side with the knees brought up to the chest.

5. Don a pair of gloves and apply KY gel to your gloved index finger.

6. Part the buttocks and examine the anus. Note the presence of any haemorrhoids, anal tags or fissures and peri-anal warts.

7. In reality, you would next ask the patient to bear down.

8. Explain to the examiner that you would inform the patient that you are now inserting a finger to examine the rectum. Insert your index finger pad first and direct it posteriorly.

9. Palpate the prostate gland anteriorly. Is the prostate gland enlarged suggesting benign prostatic hypertrophy? Is there a rock-hard nodule in the posterior lobe of the prostate gland suggestive of carcinoma? Inform the examiner of your findings.

10. Palpate for masses in the rectum.

11. Is there blood, mucus or pus on your finger?

12. Test for faecal occult blood.

13. Consider proctoscopy for the anus or sigmoidoscopy for the rectum if pathology is found.

14. Explain to the examiner that you would thank the patient for his cooperation and instruct him to get dressed.

Station 57: Answers

1. Introduce yourself to the patient and establish a rapport.

2. Ask permission to examine his chest.

3. Ask him to get undressed down to the waist.

4. Inspect the patient as he sits in front of you. What is his body habitus? Is he obese or cachectic? Is he short of breath at rest? What is his respiratory rate? Does he use any accessory muscles of respiration?

5. Inspect his chest for scars, deformities or signs of radiotherapy.

6. Examine his hands. Does he have any signs of clubbing of the fingers (bronchial carcinoma, bronchiectasis, fibrosing alveolitis, inflammatory bowel disease, infective endocarditis), cyanosis of the tips or wasting of the intrinsic muscles of the hands (Pancoast's tumour)? Does he have painful wrists (hypertrophic pulmonary osteoarthropathy clubbing, and painful wrists and ankles with characteristic X-ray changes indicative of lung malignancy. Test for asterixis. Check for pulsus paradoxus.

7. Examine the face for signs of Horner's syndrome: ptosis, enophthalmos (sunken eye), miosis and ipsilateral loss of sweating or anhydrosis. Horner's syndrome may result from invasion of the cervical sympathetic plexus at the thoracic outlet from an apical lung tumour, i.e. Pancoast's tumour.

8. Palpate the trachea. Is it midline or deviated? Is there any tracheal tug (descent with inspiration)?

9. Palpate for cervical lymphadenopathy.

10. Assess for limited chest expansion using your hands. Normal expansion should be 5 cm.

11. Palpate the chest wall and ask the patient to repeat '99'. Feel for vibration or vocal fremitus.

12. Percuss the chest and note any resonance (hyperexpanded chest or pneumothorax, dullness (consolidated lung) or stony dullness (pleural effusion).

13. Auscultate the chest. Ask the patient to breathe deeply in and out through his mouth. Note any diminished breath sounds, inspiratory or expiratory wheezes, fine or coarse crackles or pleural rub.

14. Check for vocal resonance. Auscultate as the patient repeats '99'. It should normally be muffled but increased and clearer over a consolidated lung.

15. If he has a productive cough, give the patient a specimen cup and send the sputum for culture and sensitivity.

16. Time permitting, look for the jugular venous pressure. Is it raised, i.e. > 3 cm?

17. Finally, examine the heart for signs of cor pulmonale (right heart failure due to chronic pulmonary hypertension). Signs include raised JVP, tricuspid regurgitation, ascites, hepatic enlargement and ankle oedema.

18. Thank the patient for his cooperation and instruct him to get dressed.

Station 58: Answers

1. Introduce yourself to the patient and establish a rapport.

2. Discuss the presenting complaint. Determine the severity and duration of the diarrhoea. The diarrhoea is not explosive in nature but rather small in quantity.

3. Is the diarrhoea acute or chronic in nature? She states that the problem has been intermittent over several months. The differential diagnosis for acute diarrhoea includes dietary indiscretion, pseudomembranous colitis, purgative abuse, infective causes (food poisoning or viral gastroenteritis) and traveller's diarrhoea (*E. coli*, *Giardia lamblia*, *Shigella* or *Entamoeba histolytica*). The differential diagnosis for chronic diarrhoea includes inflammatory bowel disease (Crohn's or ulcerative colitis), parasitic or fungal infections, malabsorption, irritable bowel syndrome, colonic malignancy, drugs, bowel resection, HIV infection, endocrine causes such as diabetic neuropathy, and faecal impaction in the elderly.

4. Exclude causes of acute diarrhoea. Ask about her diet. She states she dislikes vegetables. Is anyone else in the nursing home suffering from nausea/vomiting and/or diarrhoea suggestive of food poisoning? Has she travelled recently? No one else is ill and she has not travelled recently.

5. Exclude causes of chronic diarrhoea. Does she suffer from bloating and pain in the left iliac fossa, which is relieved by defecation or the passage of wind (classic for irritable bowel syndrome)? Does she suffer from fever, abdominal pain, weight loss, and/or rectal bleeding suggestive of inflammatory bowel disease? Has she had any abdominal or pelvic surgery in the past? Has she noticed blood or mucus per rectum? Has she had any changes in her bowel habits? When was her last solid stool? Is she cachectic? She is cachectic and states that her last solid stool was 2 weeks ago. She has a history of constipation and states that she feels constipated as she speaks. She is otherwise well.

6. Is there a non-gastrointestinal cause for the diarrhoea? Ask her about her prior medical history. Is she a diabetic with autonomic neuropathy and nocturnal diarrhoea or is she hyperthyroid and thyrotoxic? She denies all.

7. Ask her about her drug history. Is she taking laxatives (lactulose, magnesium sulphate), antacids, cimetidine, digoxin or thiazide diuretics? Is she on long-term antibiotics (pseudomembranous colitis)? She has been taking laxatives recently but only on a prn basis for constipation.

8. At the 30-second bell, suggest a diagnosis of faecal impaction to be confirmed by rectal examination and abdominal X-ray. Explain that to exclude anything sinister, you would like to perform an abdominal and rectal examination for masses and test for occult blood.

Station 59: Answers

1. Introduce yourself to the patient and establish a rapport.

2. Discuss the presenting complaint. Establish the severity and duration of her dysphagia. Is she dysphagic to solids and liquids? Is the nature of the problem acute or chronic? She states that she has difficulty chiefly with solids but gurgles when she drinks liquids. This problem has gradually worsened over the past months.

3. Ask key questions to determine the nature of the dysphagia. Can she tolerate fluids over solids? If yes, think stricture. If no, think motility disorders.

4. Is it difficult actually to make the swallowing movement? If yes, think bulbar palsy.

5. Is the dysphagia painful and constant? If yes, think oesophageal, pharyngeal or gastric malignancy.

6. Does the neck bulge? If yes, think pharyngeal pouch.

7. Ascertain the presence of any associated symptoms. Does she suffer from weight loss, recurrent chest infections, halitosis or food regurgitation suggestive of pharyngeal pouch? Does she suffer from anaemia, spoon-shaped fingernails (koilonychia), smooth, pale tongue and/or angular cheilosis suggestive of Plummer–Vinson syndrome or Paterson–Brown–Kelly syndrome?

8. Are there any alleviating or exacerbating factors?

9. Ask her about her prior medical history.

10. Ask about her drug history.

11. At the 30-second bell, suggest a likely diagnosis of pharyngeal pouch and the definitive investigation of choice, a barium swallow.

Station 60: Answers

1. Explain to the examiner that you would inform the nurse that you will attend to the patient immediately.

2. The examiner tells you that on arrival you find the patient in shock. He is alert but pale, diaphoretic and in excruciating abdominal pain.

3. You alert the nurse and have her bleep the registrar on call to come and assist you. She is then to return and assist you in resuscitating the patient. Meanwhile, you attend the patient. Give him 4 l min^{-1} oxygen by facemask. Insert two large-bore 14-gauge intravenous venflons and simultaneously take bloods for full blood count, urea and electrolytes, liver function tests, amylase, clotting screen and type and cross 4 units blood. Have the nurse ring for an urgent porter to collect the bloods.

4. Run Hartmann's solution into the intravenous lines.

5. Instruct the nurse to insert a Foley catheter and start a fluids' input and output chart. Instruct her to send off a sample of urine for culture and sensitivity as the patient is pyrexial. Tell the nurse that the patient is now to be kept nil by mouth.

6. Explain that you would examine the patient carefully showing particular attention to the abdominal examination. Explain that you would examine the chest to exclude a chest infection, as the patient is pyrexial. Explain that you would inspect, percuss, palpate and auscultate the abdomen. You are told that he has a rigid abdomen with generalized tenderness and guarding. Your impression is that he now has an acute abdomen with peritoneal signs.

7. Explain that you would perform a rectal examination. You are told that he has rectal bleeding.

8. He is still pyrexial and vomiting. Explain that you would insert a nasogastric tube into his stomach to prevent aspiration pneumonia.

9. Explain that you would arrange urgent portable X-rays: an upright chest X-ray to exclude free air under the diaphragm and an abdominal X-ray.

10. Explain that you would obtain an urgent surgical opinion from the surgical registrar on duty and prepare the patient for surgery.

11. Explain that you would perform a 12-lead electrocardiogram as a pre-operative measure for the patient and check that he is not reinfarcting his myocardium.

12. Explain that you would prescribe broad-spectrum intravenous antibiotics such as cefuroxime 750 mg qds and metronidazole 500 mg tds.

13. At the 30-second bell, explain that you believe that the patient most likely has acute intestinal ischaemia. The patient may have occlusion of the superior or inferior mesenteric artery from emboli post-myocardial infarction.

Station 61: Answers

1. Introduce yourself to the patient and establish a rapport.

2. Explain that you would like to conduct an examination of her cranial nerves.

3. Use smelling scents to test the ability of each nostril to detect smell. If asked by the examiner how does one determine whether the patient is malingering, answer that you would have the patient smell ammonia. The detection of this scent is carried by the trigeminal nerve and not the olfactory nerve.

4. Test the optic nerve by testing visual acuity and examining the pupils for their size, shape, symmetry, reactivity to light and accommodation.

5. Test cranial nerves III, IV and VI (oculomotor, trochlear, abducens) by checking eye movements. 'LR6, SO4 and the rest by 3' is a quick guide to remembering which eye muscles are innervated by which cranial nerves. The abducens nerve innervates the lateral rectus muscle. The superior oblique muscle is innervated by the trochlear nerve, and the rest of the eye muscles by the oculomotor nerve.

6. Asking the patient to open her mouth tests the trigeminal nerve (V). The trigeminal nerve innervated muscles of mastication.

7. To test the facial nerve (VII), ask the patient to raise her eyebrows, blow her cheeks and show you her teeth. A lower motor neuron lesion such as Bell's palsy will affect the whole of one side including the forehead. An upper motor neuron lesion will spare the forehead.

8. To test the vestibulocochlear nerve (VIII), ask the patient to repeat a whispered word in each ear (cochlear) and check for balance (Romberg or Unterburger's tests) and nystagmus. The Romberg test is conducted by asking the patient to stand with her feet together, arms by her side and her eyes shut. The Unterburger test is conducted by asking the patient to march up and down in place with her arms outstretched in front of her and her hands clasped together with her eyes shut.

9. To test the glossopharyngeal (IX) and vagal nerves (X), check the patient for a gag reflex.

10. To test the spinal accessory nerve, have the patient shrug her shoulders against resistance (trapezius muscle) and have her push your hand away with each cheek (sternomastoid muscle).

11. Finally, to test the hypoglossal nerve, ask the patient to stick out her tongue. It will deviate to the side of the lesion if present.

Station 62: Answers

1. Remark on the view in which the film was taken. 'This is a PA view of the chest.'

2. 'The obvious abnormality is the presence of cavitating secondary deposits of carcinoma of the breast in the left lung and a malignant pleural effusion in the right lung. This patient has undergone a right-sided mastectomy.'

3. Remark on the heart, mediastinum, hila, diaphragm, root of the neck and trachea, lung fields, soft tissues, and bones.

Station 63: Answers

1. Introduce yourself to the patient and establish a rapport.

2. Ask permission to examine his back.

3. Examine the patient first standing. Inspect for scars, pigmentation and spinal deformities such as kyphosis of the thoracic spine, scoliosis (lateral curvature of the spine) or lumbar lordosis. Is one knee bent suggesting nerve root tension on that side? By flexing the knee, the sciatic nerve is relaxed.

4. Palpate the spinous processes and the interspinous ligaments for any prominence or step. Localize any tenderness to the vertebrae, intervertebral tissues or paraspinous muscles.

5. Test flexion by asking the patient to attempt to touch his toes with his knees kept straight. If he straightens up by pushing on his knees, think lumbar instability. Place your fingers over two spinous processes as he bends over. If the distance between these two spinous processes in full flexion is < 5 cm, the patient is not flexing his spine but rather flexing at the hips.

6. Test extension by asking the patient to arch his spine backwards.

7. Test lateral flexion by asking the patient to bend sideways, i.e. sliding his hand down the corresponding thigh.

8. Test rotation by asking the patient to twist his torso to each side as you stabilize his pelvis by placing your hands firmly on his hips. This tests movement of the thoracic spine.

9. Assess chest expansion between maximal inspiration and expiration. The difference should be 7 cm. This tests movement at the costovertebral joints.

10. Test muscle power by asking the patient to stand up on his toes (plantarflexion) and then standing flat on his soles (dorsiflexion).

11. Ask the patient to lie on his stomach. Palpate the spine for tenderness or any bony lumps. In this position, palpate the popliteal and posterior tibial pulses, test the power of the

hamstring muscle, and test for sensation on the posterior aspect of the lower limbs.

12. Perform the femoral stretch test (for lumbar root tension) by flexing the patient's knee and lifting the hip into extension. Pain may arise in the anterior thigh and in the back.

13. Have the patient roll over onto his back (supine).

14. Perform the straight leg raising test by raising the patient's straightened leg up off the couch until the patient feels pain not only in the thigh (normal), but also in the buttock and calf (Lasegue's test). Coughing or sneezing will worsen the pain. Normally, you should be able to raise the patient's lower limb to ~80–90°. If < 45°, the straight leg raise is said to be limited and the Lasegue's sign is said to be positive. The sciatic nerve is put on further tension by dorsiflexing the foot. If pain is elicited, the sciatic stretch is positive. If straight leg raising the unaffected side causes pain on the affected side, this suggests crossed sciatic tension from a central prolapsed disc and risk to the sacral nerve roots that control bladder function.

15. Test for mobility in the hips and knees. Bending the patient's knee towards his abdomen tests flexion of the hip. If no pain is elicited, the hip joint is unaffected.

16. Test for muscle power in the lower limbs and note any muscle wasting. A tape measure can be used to compare the circumference of each thigh.

17. The femoral nerve innervates the iliopsoas (L1–3), sartorius (L2, 3) and quadriceps femoris (L2–4). Asking the patient to flex his hip with his knee flexed tests the iliopsoas muscle. Flexing the knee with the hip externally rotated tests the sartorius muscle. Extending the knee against resistance tests the quadriceps muscle.

18. The sciatic nerve innervates the hamstrings (L4, 5, S1, 2), tibialis posterior (L4, 5), tibialis anterior (L4, 5), extensor digitorum longus (L5, S1), extensor hallicus longus (L5, S1), peroneus longus and brevis (L5, S1), extensor digitorum brevis (S1), gastrocnemius (S1, 2), flexor digitorum longus (S1, 2), and the small muscles of the foot (S1, 2). Flexing the knee against resistance tests the hamstrings. Inverting a plantar-flexed foot tests the tibialis posterior. Tibialis anterior is tested by dorsiflexing the ankle. Extensor digitorum longus is tested by dorsiflexing the toes against resistance. Extensor hallucis

longus is tested by dorsiflexing the great toe against resistance. Everting the foot against resistance tests the peroneus longus and brevis. Extensor digitorum brevis is tested by dorsiflexing the hallux. Plantar-flexing the ankle tests the gastrocnemius. Flexing the terminal joints of the toes tests the flexor digitorum longus. Making the sole of the foot into a cup tests the small muscles of the foot.

19. A neurological examination of the lower limbs is performed next. Skin sensation is tested with a pin. Tendon reflexes are tested at the patellar tendon (L4) and Achilles tendon (S1), and plantars should be down-going.

20. A vascular examination of the lower limbs is performed palpating pulses.

21. A rectal examination may be required.

Station 64: Answers

1. Introduce yourself to the patient and establish a rapport.

2. Ask permission to examine his legs.

3. Ask him to undress below the waist.

4. Ask the patient to lie supine on the couch. Inspect the lower limbs for pallor or cyanosis of the skin and distribution of hair or lack thereof.

5. Ask him to raise each leg. In a normal person, the leg can be raised to 90° and the toes remain pink. In an ischaemic leg, the toes turn pale at 15–30°. A Buerger's angle of < 20° indicates severe ischaemia.

6. Next, ask the patient to sit up and hang his legs over the side of the couch. An ischaemic leg will take time to turn from white to pink and then to a flushed purple-red. The length of time for the foot to turn pink is the capillary-filling time. In severe ischaemia, the capillary filling time may be up to 30 seconds.

7. Inspect the veins of the foot as the patient is lying down again. Guttering of the veins describes veins that are collapsed and appear as pale blue gutters. Guttering of the veins occurs at 10–15° of elevation in severe ischaemia.

8. Lift the heels and inspect the undersurface and sides. Look at the malleoli and make it a point to look at the web spaces between each of the toes for sites of ulceration, trophic changes, pressure necrosis or gangrene.

9. Examine any ulcers and note the site, colour, tenderness, temperature, shape and size. A flat sloping edge indicates a superficial venous ulcer. A square-cut or punched-out edge indicates a trophic ulcer. An undermined edge indicates tuberculosis. A rolled edge suggests basal cell carcinoma and an everted edge suggests squamous cell carcinoma.

10. Palpate the lower limbs. Run the back of your fingers over the entire limb to assess for changes in temperature and at which level.

11. Check capillary refill by pressing the pulp of the toe for 2 seconds and observing the time it takes to turn pink.

12. Palpate the femoral, popliteal, posterior tibial and dorsalis pedis pulses on each side.

13. Auscultate for bruits over the course of the major arteries: abdominal aorta, iliac and femoral arteries.

14. Measure the ankle brachial Doppler index. An ankle-brachial Doppler index ratio < 0.4 indicates severe ischaemia. The ratio should normally be 1.0. Measure the blood pressure taken over the brachial artery using a hand-held Doppler and a sphygmomanometer and compare it with the blood pressure taken over the calf above the ankle.

Station 65: Answers

1. Introduce yourself to the patient and establish a rapport.

2. Ask permission to examine her legs.

3. Ask the patient to undress from the waist down but keeping her knickers on.

4. Ask the patient to stand up. Note the size and course of her varicose veins and record this on a diagram of her leg. Note any venous stars (blue patches with minute radiating veins) or ankle flares (sign of venous hypertension). Note any ankle oedema. Pay particular attention to the medial aspect of the lower leg for brown pigmentation, eczema (post-thrombotic damage) and ulceration.

5. Palpate the lower limbs along the course of the veins and note any tension. Note the presence of lipodermatosclerosis (sclerosis of the skin and subcutaneous fat with tissue death and scarring), which is a sign of chronic venous hypertension.

6. Feel at the saphenofemoral and saphenopopliteal junctions. Ask the patient to cough. A cough impulse in the groin indicates that the valves in the subcutaneous veins are incompetent.

7. Have the patient lie down. Perform the tourniquet test. Elevate one leg until all the blood has drained from the superficial veins. Place a rubber tourniquet around the upper third of the thigh. Ask the patient to stand up. If the veins only fill up above the tourniquet, this suggests an incompetent communicating vein above the tourniquet. If the veins only fill below the tourniquet, this suggests an incompetent communicating vein below the tourniquet. The tourniquet test can be repeated with the tourniquet placed below the knee. If this controls the varices, the short saphenous vein is incompetent.

8. The Trendelenburg test is performed by elevating one leg until the blood has drained from the superficial veins and then digitally compressing the saphenofemoral junction in the groin to prevent retrograde filling. The patient is then asked to stand up with your hand still compressing the saphenofemoral junction to test the competence of the long saphenous vein. If the veins remain empty, the long saphenous vein is incompetent.

9. Test for a palpable percussion impulse by placing the fingers of one hand lightly over the lower limit of the visible veins and tapping the upper limit. If a percussion wave is transmitted, this suggests an incompetent valve.

10. Auscultate over clusters of veins with the patient lying down to exclude an arteriovenous fistula.

Station 66: Answers

1. Introduce yourself to the patient and establish a rapport.

2. Ask permission to examine his feet.

3. Inspect the feet for deformities such as pes cavus, claw toes, Charcot's joints (a painless, swollen, disorganized joint caused from excessive movement and loss of sensation at the joint), loss of transverse arch and rocker-bottom sole.

4. Inspect the feet for both neuropathic and ischaemic ulcers. A neuropathic or trophic ulcer usually occurs on the soles of the foot of patients with diabetic peripheral neuritis. They are deep, painless, penetrating ulcers found over pressure points. The surrounding tissues have a normal blood supply but are less sensitive to pain. Ischaemic ulcers are painful and discharge a thin serous exudate. There may be a history of minor trauma to the area. The ulcer shows no signs of healing and often gets larger and deeper. They are usually located over the tips of the toes or at pressure points. The surrounding tissues are cold and ischaemic. The base may contain grey-yellow sloughing tissue with a punched-out edge. Note whether the ulcer is infected.

5. Perform a vascular examination. Palpate the feet for temperature and check peripheral pulses. Use a Doppler if you have difficulty detecting the pulses. Check capillary refill time.

6. Perform a neurological examination. Test for sensation. The diabetic foot will have a stocking distribution of sensory loss. The ankle jerk reflexes are often absent.

7. Examine the movement of the ankle joint and feet. A Charcot ankle and foot caused by diabetic neuropathy will have limited movement.

8. Thank the patient for his cooperation.

Station 67: Answers

1. Introduce yourself to the patient and establish a rapport.

2. Ask permission to examine her legs.

3. Ask her to walk up and down before you and examine her gait. Ask her to walk on her toes and then heels.

4. Inspect her legs for signs of neuropathic ulcers or joints, muscle wasting or fasciculations.

5. Assess the sensation in the lower limbs using a cotton ball for light touch and a vibrating 128 Hx tuning fork for vibration (posterior column–dorsal column/medial leminiscus pathways). Assess two-point discrimination (normal is 2 cm on the soles of the feet). Assess the anterolateral spinothalamic tracts by using a pin for pinprick sensation and temperature discrimination.

6. Be aware of the sensory dermatomes for the lower limb. A rough guide is as follows: L1 covers the hips and groin. S2 and 3 cover the genital region. L2 covers the anterior thigh. L3 covers the lower anterior thigh and medial patella. L4 covers the lateral patella, shin and medial leg. L5 covers the lateral leg and four medial toes anteriorly and S1 the posterior calf, the little toe anteriorly, and the sole of the foot and toes posteriorly. Posteriorly, S2 covers the posterior thigh with L3 laterally and medially, and S3 covers the peri-anal region.

7. Be aware that the branches of the sciatic nerve include the lateral cutaneous nerve of the calf, superficial and deep peroneal nerves, sural, and medial plantar nerves. Lesions of the sciatic nerve (L4–S2) affect muscles below the knee and sensation below the knee laterally.

8. Be aware that a lesion of the lateral popliteal nerve (L4–S2) leads to equinovarus with an inability to dorsiflex the foot and sensory loss over the dorsum of the foot.

9. Be aware that a lesion of the tibial nerve (S1–3) leads to calcaneovarus with inability to stand on tiptoe or evert the foot and sensory loss over the sole of the foot.

10. Assess the motor system next. Test for power (hip flexion, ankle dorsiflexion) and tone.

11. Muscle weakness is graded 0–5. Grade 0 is no contraction; 1, a flicker of a contraction; 2, active movement with gravity eliminated; 3, active movement against gravity; 4, active movement against gravity and resistance; and 5, normal power.

12. Signs of an upper motor neuron lesion include spasticity (hypertonia in the extensors of the legs), paralysis or weakness in the flexors of the legs, and ankle clonus elicited by flexing the patient's ankle. Signs of a lower motor neuron lesion include muscle wasting, fasciculations, decreased or absent reflexes and muscle weakness.

13. Check the patellar tendon reflex and ankle jerk reflex. Check that plantars are down-going. If they are extensor plantars (up-going), think upper motor neuron lesion.

14. Thank the patient for her cooperation.

Station 68: Answers

1. Introduce yourself to the patient and establish a rapport.

2. Hand her the peak flow meter with the fitted cardboard attachment.

3. Ask her to take deep breaths in and out. Ask her then to hold a deep breath and blow as hard and as fast as she can into the peak flow meter. Make sure she has maintained a proper seal with her mouth.

4. Read the peak flow meter.

5. Give her another attempt and record the best reading.

6. Ask her for her height. She states that she is 5 foot 3 inches. Know how to convert feet to metres: 1 inch = 2.54 cm. She stands 1.6 m tall. As she is only 22, she should achieve a peak expiratory flow rate (PEFR) of just over 400 l min^{-1}. At age 40, she should achieve a PEFR of 400 l min^{-1}, and by age 60, this falls to 350 l min^{-1}.

7. An average young man standing 1.85 metres tall (or 6 foot 1 inch) should achieve a PEFR of 650 l min^{-1} and a young man standing 5 feet 7 inches tall should achieve a PEFR of 600 l min^{-1}. These measurements fall by 50 l min^{-1} by age 40 and by 100 l min^{-1} by age 60.

8. If her present PEFR falls below her normal PEFR, she will need to increase her dose of inhalers during her bout of chest infection.

9. Thank the patient for her cooperation.

Station 69: Answers

1. Remark on the view in which the film was taken. 'This is a PA view of the chest.'

2. 'This patient has miliary tuberculosis.' If asked what else would you examine besides the chest, reply: 'I would wish to examine the patient's retina looking for tuberculosis and the patient's legs looking for erythema nodosum.'

3. Remark on the heart, mediastinum, hila, diaphragm, root of the neck and trachea, lung fields, soft tissues, and bones.

Station 70: Answers

1. Determine which view the film was taken. 'This is a PA view of the chest.'

2. 'The obvious abnormality is a right-sided tension pneumothorax with collapse of the right lung and deviation of the trachea to the opposite side.'

3. Comment on the heart, mediastinum, hila, diaphragm, root of the neck, lung fields, soft tissues, and bones.

Station 71: Answers

1. Explain to the examiner that you would introduce yourself to the patient. Do not address the manikin.

2. Explain to the examiner that you would ask permission of the patient to examine the back of his eyes.

3. Explain to the examiner that you would darken the room and ask the patient to focus on an object in the far corner and not look directly into the ophthalmoscope.

4. Assess the lens for cataract (opacity), which is a common eye finding in diabetics. There should be an absence of red reflex if present and an inability to assess the fundus.

5. Once cataract has been excluded, assess the iris for rubeosis (new vessel formation), which puts the patient at risk for glaucoma.

6. Assess the retina. In the examination, a slide may be projected. Background diabetic retinopathy (non-proliferative) appears as exudates, haemorrhages and micro-aneurysms. Micro-aneurysms leak plasma and lipids seen as hard exudates. Soft exudates are sites of small retinal infarcts.

7. In proliferative diabetic retinopathy, common in IDDM after 5–20 years, there is new vessel formation near the optic disc and fibrosis. The patient is then at risk for haemorrhage, retinal detachment and ultimately blindness.

8. Repeat the examination on the opposite side.

9. Explain to the examiner, that you would thank the patient for his cooperation.

Station 72: Answers

1. Determine which view the film was taken. 'This is a PA view of the chest.'

2. 'The obvious abnormality is a fracture of the right clavicle.'

3. Comment on the heart, mediastinum, hila, diaphragm, root of the neck and trachea, lung fields, soft tissues, and bones.

Station 73: Answers

1. Explain that you would initially dry the amniotic fluid covering the infant and place her under a preheated warmer. Take the baby manikin, dry her, wrap her in warm towels and position her on her back. Avoid hyperextension or flexion of the neck as this may obstruct the airway.

2. Suction the mouth before the nose and stimulate the baby by flicking the soles of her feet.

3. Determine the patient's Apgar score (heart rate, respiratory effort, muscle tone, reflex/irritability, colour).

4. Apply 100% oxygen if the respirations are shallow or slow. Keep the mask slightly off to the side as the oxygen currents are cold. Reassess the baby after 15 seconds.

5. If the baby is apnoeic, with a heart rate < 100 or has persistent cyanosis, apply bag-valve mask ventilation using a disposable blue 450–70-ml bag. Make sure the yellow cap is removed (pop-off valve) and ventilate at 40–60 breaths per minute. Observe for bilateral chest expansion and adequate colour, and ausculate for bilateral breath sounds.

6. Re-evaluate the baby after 30 seconds. You are told by the examiner that the heart rate has now dropped to 55. Perform chest compressions with two thumbs or two fingers depressing the sternum by one-third. Perform chest compressions to ventilation at a ratio of 3:1 or a chest compression rate of 120 min^{-1}. Stop once the heart rate is > 80.

7. You are told by the examiner that the baby is pink, breathing spontaneously and the heart rate is > 100. Cease resuscitation protocol.

8. Determine the baby's 5-minute Apgar score.

Station 74: Answers

This is a favourite PLAB 2 OSCE station, and you may also be asked to perform an abdominal examination.

1. Introduce yourself to the patient and establish a rapport.

2. Obtain a history of the presenting complaint.

3. Ask her to describe the pain, its site, character, radiation, intensity and frequency of attacks. She explains that the pain was epigastric but now is localized to the right upper abdomen. The pain is colicky in nature.

4. Establish whether the pain is acute or chronic and persistent or intermittent in nature. She explains that the attacks last for up to 5 days and have been getting worse.

5. Establish any exacerbating factors or relieving factors. She states that it is worse after eating. Ask her about her diet. She admits to eating a fry up for breakfast and fish and chips for supper. She takes painkillers for the pain.

6. Establish any associated symptoms. She complains lately of nausea and vomiting. She has come in today because she is feverish and the pain is severe.

7. Ask her about her medical history. She explains she has only been in hospital when she had her four children by vaginal delivery. She suffers from a hiatus hernia.

8. Ask her about her drug history. She is on the combined oral contraceptive pill.

9. At the 30-second bell, suggest a diagnosis of previous biliary colic now presenting as acute cholecystitis.

Station 75: Answers

1. Explain to the examiner that you would introduce yourself to the patient.

2. Explain to the examiner that you would ask permission of the patient to examine the back of his eyes.

3. Explain to the examiner that you would darken the room and ask the patient to focus on an object at the back of the room.

4. Examine the lens for cataracts.

5. Examine the iris for rubeosis (new vessel formation).

6. Examine the retina. You may be shown a slide of the retinal findings. Look for signs of vascular disease: copper-wiring of arteries (grade I), arteriovenous nipping (II), flame and blot haemorrhages and cotton wool exudates (III) and for papilloedema (IV).

7. Repeat the examination on the opposite side.

8. Explain to the examiner that you would thank the patient for her cooperation.

Station 76: Answers

This is a favourite PLAB 2 OSCE station!

1. Introduce yourself to the patient and establish a rapport.

2. Explain to him that he is being discharged home today. Explain that he has suffered a heart attack but has recovered well.

3. Ask him if he would like a sick certificate, as he will be off work for 3 months.

4. Advise him to take it easy at home and avoid strenuous activity. He should not drive for the next 3 months.

5. Inform him of the known risk factors for heart disease. Advise him to stop smoking and reduce his alcohol intake. If he is obese, advise him to lose weight and cut out salt from his diet. If his cholesterol level is high, advise him to cut down on fatty foods.

6. Inform him that he has four medications to take home with him. The GTN tablet is to be taken on an as needed basis. Should he suffer angina (chest pains), he is to place one tablet under his tongue and close his mouth. If the pain does not subside, he should repeat the tablet (up to 1 mg total) or three tablets over 10 minutes. If the pain persists, he should call for an ambulance to take him to Casualty.

7. Aspirin is to be taken once a day. Aspirin should thin his blood and help prevent future clot formation in his coronary vessels. The side-effects of taking aspirin include risk of epistaxis and heartburn. If he should experience a heavy nosebleed that does not abate with pressure over the nares, he should see his GP immediately or call for an ambulance to take him to Casualty. If he suffers from heartburn, he should see his GP and take gaviscon or antacids in the meantime.

8. The gliclazide is for his diabetes. The side-effects are mild gastrointestinal upset and headache, but these side-effects are mild and infrequent. He should have his blood glucose monitored by his GP and attend Diabetic Clinic for annual review.

9. The ternormin tablet or atenolol is a β-blocker, which means that it will slow his heart rate. It is to be taken to prevent angina (chest pain). He is to take one tablet twice a day. The reported side-effects of tenormin include bradycardia, hypotension, fatigue, sleep disorders and intermittent claudication. Explain these side-effects in layman's terms. However, explain that these are only reported side-effects and do not occur in every individual.

10. Explain that he will be sent a follow-up appointment to the Cardiology Clinic for 4–6 week's time.

11. Explain that his GP will receive a copy of his hospital discharge paper.

12. Ask him if he has any questions. Ask him whether he has understood your instructions or needs clarification.

13. Thank the patient for listening.

Station 77: Answers

1. Introduce yourself to the patient and establish a rapport.

2. Explain that she has been diagnosed with epilepsy but is well enough to be discharged home. Explain that epilepsy means seizures or fits and that often the cause is unknown.

3. Explain that she has been started on an anticonvulsant medication called phenytoin at 300 mg od to prevent future seizures. Explain that she must not stop the medication unless she is advised to do so by her GP. State that possible side-effects of this drug include rashes, gum hypertrophy, folate deficiency, polyneuropathy and osteomalacia, but most are associated with chronic use.

4. Explain that her serum level of phenytoin will be monitored to ensure that she has attained a therapeutic level of the drug in her blood stream.

5. Ask her if she is taking a combined oral contraceptive pill. Advise her that the combined pill is less effective when taken in conjunction with certain anti-epileptic medication such as phenytoin, and that she should see her GP to change her pill to one containing higher does of oestrogen and progestogen.

6. Explain that the social consequences of epilepsy include a ban on driving if she has suffered more than one seizure. To obtain a UK driving licence, she has to have been seizure-free while awake for 2 years before the issue of a licence. If her attacks occur in her sleep, she must have been seizure-free for 3 years before the issue of a licence.

7. Explain that the laws are stricter for Public Service Vehicle or Heavy Goods Vehicle licences and that she will not be issued one.

8. Advise her to wear an identity bracelet to alert persons that she suffers from epilepsy in case she collapses.

9. Advise the patient to avoid swimming alone or engaging in risky sports alone.

10. Advise the patient to leave her bathroom door unlocked and to take shallow baths.

11. Inform the patient that she will be sent a follow-up outpatient appointment for 4–6 weeks.

12. Inform the patient that the GP will receive a copy of her hospital discharge paper and that he will be capable of managing her care.

13. Ask the patient if she has any questions. Ask her if she has understood everything that has been explained to her or whether she needs clarification.

Station 78: Answers

1. Introduce yourself to the patient and establish a rapport.

2. Ask her about her presenting complaint. Establish the duration of symptoms and the length of each episode. It may help to discuss the episodes with a family witness. Is each episode preceded by an aura (focal seizure)? Does she utter a cry and fall? Has she bitten her tongue or been found incontinent of urine or faeces? Was this followed by a brief muscle convulsion and hours lying comatose (tonic-clonic seizure)? Has she experienced *déjà vu* or any visual hallucinations (temporal lobe seizures)?

3. Determine the possible aetiological and precipitating factors.

4. Ask the patient if she has a family history of epilepsy. About 30% of patients will have a first-degree relative with a history of epilepsy.

5. Ask the patient if she has suffered any recent head trauma or surgery. Epilepsy may occur within the first week or years later.

6. Obtain a drug history from the patient. Does she drink alcohol or partake of recreational drugs? Amphetamines and alcohol abuse may precipitate seizures. Is she on medication? Tricyclic antidepressants may provoke a fit in a patient with a low seizure threshold.

7. Be aware of the causes of epilepsy: encephalitis, chronic meningitis (tuberculosis), cerebral abscess, intracranial masses, metabolic derangements, etc.

8. Exclude other causes of recurrent attacks of loss of consciousness such as vasovagal attacks, carotid sinus syndrome, transient ischaemic attacks, postural hypotension in patients with autonomic neuropathy or on ganglion-blocking antihypertensives, hypoglycaemia, cardiac arrhythmias and effort syncope.

9. Ask the patient whether she experiences any warning signs such as palpitations (cardiac arrhythmias), hunger and sweating (hypoglycaemia), or light-headedness with circumoral and peripheral tingling (hyperventilation)?

10. At the 30-second bell, offer a diagnosis of epilepsy.

Station 79: Answers

This is a favourite PLAB 2 OSCE station!

1. Introduce yourself to the patient and establish a rapport.

2. Note the appearance, behaviour and demeanour of the patient.

3. Ask her about her symptoms. How long have these symptoms been bothering her? Since the baby was born? Psychiatric blues usually begin on days 2–3 after delivery.

4. Does she suffer from lowered mood or mood swings, insomnia, lack of self-esteem, anxiety, or tearfulness? Yes to all of the above. The actor starts to behave in an anxious, loud and aggressive manner.

5. Does she fear she will harm or neglect her baby? Yes. Ask her to elaborate. She is afraid to be alone with the baby and sometimes feels an urge to place a pillow over the baby's face and suffocate it.

6. Determine her risk factors. Is she > 30 years of age? Yes.

7. Has she been pregnant before and, if so, has she suffered previous postpartum psychiatric illness? She states she has been pregnant before.

8. Has she had any miscarriages or stillbirths? She has had one stillbirth.

9. Did she suffer depression during this pregnancy? Yes.

10. Was the pregnancy or delivery difficult or traumatic? Yes, the labour was prolonged, resulting in an emergency Caesarean section.

11. Has she been breast-feeding for the past 3 months? Yes.

12. Does she have a history of mood disorder or any psychiatric illness? No.

13. Does she suffer from premenstrual tension? Yes.

14. Does she have any marital problems? Yes.

15. Does she feel she has lack of support, i.e. lack of social contact? Yes.

16. Clinical post-natal depression affects 5% of women. Frank psychosis affects 0.3% and is potentially life threatening to the mother and baby. If the patient has post-natal depression, then offer counselling, an increase in social support and anti-depressant medication.

17. If you determine that the patient has psychosis, exhibiting symptoms of rejection of the baby, confusion and/or delusion, admit the patient to the Mother–Baby Unit of the psychiatric ward and ensure 24-hour supervision. Start the patient on antipsychotic medication after consultation with your registrar or consultant.

18. In this station, the mother poses a threat to the well-being of her child and should be admitted with her baby to the Mother–Baby Unit.

Station 80: Answers

This is a favourite PLAB 2 OSCE station!

The following answer comes from the *Advanced Trauma Life Support Manual* published by the American College of Surgeons.

1. **Obtain AMPLE history** of the injury-producing event from the patient, family or prehospital personnel.

2. **Head and maxillofacial: assessment.** Inspect and palpate the entire head and face for lacerations, contusions, fractures and thermal injury. Re-evaluate the pupils. Re-evaluate the level of consciousness. Assess the eyes for haemorrhage, penetrating injury, visual acuity, dislocation of the lens and presence of contact lens. Evaluate cranial nerve function. Inspect the ears and nose for cerebrospinal fluid.

3. **Head and maxillofacial: management.** Maintain the airway and continue ventilation and oxygenation as indicated. Control haemorrhage. Prevent secondary brain injury. Remove contact lenses.

4. **Cervical spine and neck: assessment.** Inspect for signs of blunt and penetrating injury, tracheal deviation and use of accessory muscles. Palpate for tenderness, deformity, swelling, subcutaneous emphysema and tracheal deviation. Auscultate the carotid arteries for bruits. Obtain a lateral cervical spine X-ray.

5. **Cervical spine and neck: management.** Maintain adequate in-line immobilization and protection of the spine.

6. **Chest: assessment.** Inspect the anterior, lateral, and posterior chest wall for signs of blunt and penetrating injury, use of accessory muscles, and bilateral respiratory excursions. Auscultate the anterior chest wall and posterior bases for bilateral breath sounds and heart sounds. Palpate the entire chest wall for evidence of blunt and penetrating injury, subcutaneous emphysema, tenderness, and crepitation. Percuss for evidence of dullness or hyper-resonance. Obtain a chest X-ray.

7. **Chest: management.** Tube thoracostomy as indicated and attached the chest tube to an underwater seal drainage device. Dress an open chest wound. Pericardiocentesis as indicated.

8. **Abdomen: assessment.** Inspect the anterior and posterior abdomen for signs of blunt and penetrating injury, and internal bleeding. Auscultate for bowel sounds. Percuss the abdomen to elicit subtle rebound tenderness. Palpate the abdomen for tenderness, involuntary muscle guarding and rebound tenderness. Obtain an X-ray of the pelvis. Perform diagnostic peritoneal lavage, if indicated.

9. **Abdomen: management.** Transfer the patient to theatre, if indicated. Apply a pneumatic antishock garment, if indicated.

10. **Perineum/rectum/vagina: assessment.** Inspect the perineum for contusions, haematomas, lacerations and bleeding at the urethral meatus. Inspect the rectum for the presence of blood, anal sphincter tone, bowel wall integrity, bony fragments and position of the prostate. Do not insert a Foley catheter if the patient has a high-riding prostate! Inspect the vagina for presence of blood or lacerations.

11. **Musculoskeletal: assessment.** Inspect the upper and lower extremities for evidence of blunt and penetrating injury, including contusions, haematomas, lacerations and deformities. Palpate the upper and lower extremities for tenderness, crepitation, abnormal movement and sensation. Palpate all peripheral pulses. Assess the pelvis for evidence of fracture and haemorrhage. Palpate the thoracic and lumbar spine for evidence of blunt and penetrating injury, including contusions, lacerations, tenderness, deformity and sensation. Evaluate the pelvic X-ray for evidence of a fracture. Obtain X-rays of suspected fracture sites.

12. **Musculoskeletal: management.** Apply or readjust appropriate splinting devices for extremity fractures as indicated. Maintain immobilization of the patient's thoracic and lumbar spine. Apply the pneumatic antishock garment if indicated. Administer tetanus immunization. Administer medications as indicated.

13. **Neurologic: assessment.** Re-evaluate the pupils and level of consciousness. Determine the GCS Score. Evaluate the upper and lower extremities for motor and sensory responses. Evaluate for evidence of paralysis or paresis.

14. **Neurologic: management.** Continue ventilation and oxygenation. Maintain adequate immobilization of the entire patient.

Station 81: Answers

This is a favourite PLAB 2 OSCE station!

1. Explain to the examiner that you would attend the patient immediately. You are told that on arrival she is drowsy and confused. You would resuscitate the patient. With the aid of the nurse, administer 100% oxygen by facemask and insert two large-bore intravenous cannulas for administration of intravenous fluids such as Hartmann's solution to cover for hypovolaemic shock. Simultaneously, take blood for full blood count, clotting, urea and electrolytes, and type and cross two units. Obtain an arterial blood gas to aid in exclusion of a postoperative pulmonary embolus. Have the nurse recheck her vital signs: temperature, blood pressure and pulse. Insert a Foley catheter to monitor her hourly input and output of fluids.

2. Obtain as much history from the nurse and the patient. Did the patient complain of pain in the chest or abdomen? Is she a diabetic? If so, what is her fingerstick glucose? Does she have a history of heart disease? Review her drug chart. The patient has now lost consciousness.

3. Examine the patient thoroughly from head to toe. Check the pupils for asymmetry, response to light and accommodation. Auscultate the chest to exclude postoperative pneumonia or worsening congestive heart failure and the heart. Examine the abdomen for peritoneal signs to exclude internal bleeding. On examination, the abdomen is tense with no bowel sounds. Also, perform a rectal exam for blood.

4. The examiner will ask you what you would like him to do. There is no registrar at your district general hospital. Inform him that you would like him to come urgently and review the patient with a view to taking her back to theatre for an exploratory laparotomy and proceed.

5. The examiner tells you that it will take him an hour to get to the hospital. Inform the examiner that you would prepare her for theatre and obtain a verbal consent from her next of kin over the telephone. Explain that you would inform theatres and the anaesthetist on call.

6. Inform the examiner that you would perform an urgent 12-lead electrocardiogram to exclude acute myocardial infarction

or pulmonary embolus, and that you would arrange an urgent portable chest X-ray to exclude lung pathology and free air under the diaphragm and an abdominal X-ray.

7. The haemoglobin comes back as 7.8 g dl^{-1}. Her blood pressure is now 60 palpable. Explain that you would transfuse 2 units blood as soon as possible and type and cross a further 4 units for theatre. You would inform the anaesthetist on call of the urgency of the situation.

8. The examiner informs you that the consultant is held up in traffic. You explain that you would take the patient to theatre and open the abdomen. If a bleeding vessel is found, you will attempt to clamp and ligate the bleeding vessel to buy the consultant time to arrive and take over.

9. The examiner tells you that a ligature had slipped off the splenic artery and that you have saved her life.

Station 82: Answers

This is a favourite PLAB 2 OSCE station!

1. Identify yourself to Mrs James on the telephone.

2. Ask her how you can help her? She explains that her daughter has a high temperature, has not been sleeping and complains of right earache. She thinks her daughter has an ear infection. She has tried giving Calpol to settle the temperature and pain, but to no avail. She explains that her GP cannot see her until next week. Should she bring her daughter to Casualty today? She has heard a lot in the news about meningitis. Should she be concerned for her daughter?

3. Ask her if she has taken the daughter's temperature and, if so, how high it is. She tells you it is 40°C. Inform the mother that the symptoms and signs of meningitis include fever, vomiting, headache, neck stiffness, photophobia, anorexia, irritability, confusion and lethargy. Has the child exhibited any of these symptoms or signs? Has the child had a recent chest infection? Does the child have a rash that does not blanch to pressure? The mother denies all except for the fever and right ear pain.

4. Reassure the mother that the child is unlikely to have meningitis, but as the child's temperature is so high, she should bring the child to Paediatric Casualty for assessment. The child may have an ear infection that will need to be treated with antibiotics. The child can also be assessed to exclude other causes for her pyrexia and be treated accordingly, as Calpol has had little effect.

5. Ask the mother if she has any further questions.

Station 83: Answers

1. Introduce yourself to the patient and establish a rapport.

2. Note the patient's non-verbal behaviour. Is she dressed all in black? Does she have a hunched, self-hugging posture and express little eye contact? Is she tearful with downcast eyes?

3. Ask the patient how she is? Listen to her attentively and repeat key points to assure her that you are listening. She informs you that her husband has recently passed away from prostate cancer and that ever since she has felt low and tearful. She has lost her appetite and interest in life. Her chief concern is that she has trouble sleeping and has come to you for sleeping tablets.

4. Ask her about her present circumstances. Does she have contact with close friends and relatives?

5. Ask her about her drug history. Is she on medication? Does she drink alcohol? Has she taken sleeping tablets before? If so, determine whether she may be addicted to benzodiazepines?

6. Ask her about her past. Does she have a history of depression? What is she normally like? What is her baseline premorbid personality?

7. Ask her about any family history of depression or mental illness?

8. Perform a Mental State Examination. Make notes under verbal and non-verbal behaviour.

9. Note her mood and whether she has thought of harming herself or others.

10. Note any abnormal beliefs (delusions) or ideas.

11. Note any unusual experiences or hallucinations.

12. Is she oriented to time, place, and person?

13. Test her short- and long-term memory. Ask her to recall a name and address after 5 minutes. Ask her who her MP is or who was elected Prime Minister?

14. Test her concentration. Have her recite the months of the year backwards.

15. Ask her to clarify what she means by the sentence that she has no interest in life. If you determine that she is at risk of self-harm, suggest that you admit her to the psychiatric ward. If you determine that she is depressed, suggest consultation with your registrar and starting her on an antidepressant.

16. The examiner will ask you whether you would prescribe sleeping tablets for this woman. Answer that if she has no suicidal ideation or prior history of benzodiazepine addiction, that you would prescribe a short course of low-dose sleeping tablets, but that you would suggest she receive bereavement counselling and be started on an antidepressant.

Station 84: Answers

1. Introduce yourself to the patient and establish a rapport.

2. Ask questions about the presenting complaint. Determine the duration of the fever. Is it acute or chronic? Intermittent or persistent in nature?

3. Ask questions geared towards narrowing the list of causes for fever. Has he been travelling abroad recently? No.

4. Has he recently been immunized? No.

5. Has he come into contact with animals or ill persons? No.

6. Does he have any bites, cuts or rashes? He has a blue-red rash on his nose and cheeks.

7. Does he have a chest infection? Cough, sputum production, shortness of breath? He complains of cough and malaise.

8. Does he have any lumps on his body? Enlarged lymph nodes? He has enlarged neck nodes and painful nodules on his anterior shins.

9. Does he suffer from night sweats or weight loss? No.

10. Does he have any nausea, vomiting, anorexia, abdominal pain or diarrhoea? No.

11. Does he suffer from arthritis? Yes in his hands. He has sausage-like digits.

12. Does he take any medication? Does he suffer from itching? No.

13. Has he recently had an operation? No.

14. Explain that the differential diagnosis for fever of unknown origin includes infection (abscess, tuberculosis, granulomatoma, parasites, bacteria, infective endocarditis, viruses and HIV-related infections), neoplasms (lymphoma, tumours and leukaemia), connective tissue diseases (rheumatoid arthritis, SLE, PAN, etc.), and others, such as drug reaction, sarcoid,

pulmonary emboli, inflammatory bowel disease, intracranial pathology and factitious causes.

15. At the 30-second bell, suggest a diagnosis of sarcoidosis based on the patient's symptoms of signs of fever, cough, malaise, lymphadenopathy, lupus pernio, erythema nodosum, arthralgia, dactylitis and his origin. Recommend a chest X-ray to assess for bilateral hilar lymphadenopathy and diffuse reticular shadowing.

Station 85: Answers

1. Introduce yourself to the patient and establish a rapport.

2. Reassure the patient and obtain a history. He informs you that the chest pain is unbearable and has lasted for almost an hour. He is sweaty, distressed and clammy.

3. Give the patient oxygen via facemask or nasal cannula at 4–6 l min^{-1}.

4. Site a large-bore iv cannula and take bloods for cardiac enzymes (troponin I, creatinine kinase, AST, LDH), full blood count, urea and electrolytes, and Group and Save.

5. Perform a 12-lead electrocardiogram and attach the patient to continuous ECG monitoring. Look for ST elevation, T inversion and Q waves. Confirm a diagnosis of acute myocardial infarction (MI).

6. Give diamorphine 5 mg iv for analgesia in conjunction with an antiemetic, cyclizine 50 mg iv or metoclopramide 10 mg iv. Repeat diamorphine in 5 minutes, if indicated.

7. Give glyceryl trinitrate iv – 10–200 mcg min^{-1}.

8. Give low molecular weight heparin subcutaneously tds as prophylaxis against deep vein thrombosis (DVT).

9. Arrange for a portable chest X-ray to exclude aortic dissection and congestive heart failure.

10. Admit the patient to the Coronary Care Unit.

11. Start antithrombolytic therapy ideally within 3–6 hours of an acute MI with streptokinase or TPA as long as there are no patient contraindications. Contraindications to antifibrinolytic therapy include CVA or active bleeding in the past 2 months, SBP > 200 mmHg, surgery or trauma in the past 10 days, bleeding disorder, proliferative diabetic retinopathy, or previous streptokinase treatment in the last 5 days to 1 year. The dose for SK is 1.5 million units in 100 ml 0.9% saline ivi over 1 hour with aspirin (160 mg od).

12. If the troponin I (new cardiac enzyme) level returns as high, suspicion should be high for MI. Proceed urgently to an inpatient angiogram and then on to urgent percutaneous transluminal coronary angioplasty as indicated.

Station 86: Answers

1. Introduce yourself to the patient and establish a rapport.

2. Ask permission to examine his legs.

3. Inspect the patient as a whole. Look for signs of facial hemiparesis, thyroid disease, muscle wasting, muscle fasciculation, etc. Is he using a walking cane or is he wheel chair bound?

4. Inspect both legs. Does he have tibia bowing, pes cavus, asymmetry of the legs (polio), generalized proximal muscle wasting (polymyositis), anterior thigh wasting (diabetic amyotrophy), generalized disuse atrophy (upper motor neurone disease such as severe spastic paraparesis) or muscle fasciculation (upper motor neurone disease)?

5. Test the muscle tone in each leg by passively moving it at the hip and knee joints.

6. Test the power as follows:
   - Ask the patient to lift his leg up and try to stop you from pushing it down (L1, 2).
   - Ask the patient to bend his knee and stop you from straightening it (L5, S1, 2).
   - Ask the patient to keep his knee bent and now push out straight against your hand (L3, 4).
   - Ask the patient to bend his foot down and try to push your hand away (S1).
   - Ask the patient to cock up his foot and point his toes to the ceiling. Now try to stop you from pushing his foot down (L4, 5).

7. Test coordination. Ask the patient to put his heel just below the opposite knee and run it all the way down his shin and then up again until you tell him to stop.

8. Test the deep tendon reflexes for the knee (L3, 4) and the ankle (S1, 2). If the reflexes are brisk, try to demonstrate ankle clonus.

9. Test the Babinski or plantar reflex by running the opposite end of your reflex hammer up the lateral side of the sole and turning inwards towards the big toe when you reach a point just below the little toe. An up-going (toe) plantar response suggests upper motor neurone disease.

10. The full neurological examination includes test for sensation in dermatomes L2–S1 for each leg. This is performed by dabbing cotton wool (light touch) and using a pin (pinprick) on the outer thigh (L2), inner thigh (L3), inner calf (L4), outer calf (L5), medial foot (L5) and lateral foot (S1). Check also for stocking-glove distribution of sensory loss with peripheral neuropathy. Vibration is tested on the medial malleoli, and joint position sense in the great toes. Ask the patient to close his eyes and tell you if you have moved his great toe up or down. Hold the side of the great toe as you move the toe.

11. This is then followed by test of gait (ordinary gait, walking heel to toe to exclude ataxia, walking on his toes and then his heels).

12. Finally, perform the Romberg test. If positive, think sensory ataxia such as subacute combined degeneration or tabes dorsalis).

13. For this station, note the findings in the following format:

N.S.: alert and orientated
uses crutches

P.N.S.: upper limbs – NAD
lower limbs – right quadriceps wasting
inspection – talipes equinovarus bilaterally

		R	L
Tone:		↑	↑
	°clonus bilaterally		
Power:	Hip F/E	4+	5
	Knee F/E	4+	5
	Ankle F/E	4+	5
Coordination:		NAD	NAD
Reflexes:	Knee	+++	+++
	Ankle	+++	+++
	Plantar reflex	↑	↑

Station 87: Answers

The following answer is obtained from the *Advanced Trauma Life Support Manual* published by the American College of Surgeons.

1. Explain to the examiner that the initial trauma assessment begins with the primary survey.

2. **Airway with cervical spine control**: explain to the examiner that you would assess the airway for patency. Inspect for foreign bodies in the airway. Inspect for mandibular, maxillofacial, or tracheal/laryngeal fractures. Perform the chin lift or jaw thrust manoeuvre. If the patient is unconscious or has no gag reflex, use an oropharyngeal airway to maintain the airway.

3. Be wary of cervical spine injury. Great care must be taken to prevent excessive movement of the patient's neck until the cervical spine has been cleared. The cervical spine should be cleared by both a neurological examination and a cross-table lateral cervical spine X-ray. The latter should include a clear view of the C-7 to T-1 interspace.

4. **Breathing**: expose the chest to assess ventilation. Auscultate for equal, bilateral breath sounds. Percuss for the presence of air or blood in the chest. Inspect and palpate to assess injuries to the chest wall. Exclude tension pneumothorax, flail chest with pulmonary contusion, open pneumothorax and massive haemothorax. If the patient is suspected to have any of the above, treat immediately.

5. Administer supplemental oxygen by mask/reservoir device.

6. **Circulation with haemorrhage control**: assess the patient's level of consciousness, skin colour and pulse (carotid or femoral). Severe haemorrhage is identified and controlled by direct manual pressure on the wound. Tourniquets should not be used as they crush tissues and cause distal ischaemia. If the patient is hypovolaemic, think intra-abdominal or -thoracic injury, fractures of the pelvis or long bones, penetrating injuries with vascular involvement or external haemorrhage from any source.

7. Management includes establishing two large-calibre intravenous catheters (14 or 16 gauge). If the patient has poor

venous access, consider other peripheral line access, cutdowns or central venous lines. Blood should be taken for full blood count, clotting, urea and electrolytes, liver function tests, amylase, β-HCG (in child-bearing females), and type and cross-match 4 units. Hartmann's solution or Ringer's lactate solution is the preferred initial bolus infusion. Hypovolaemic shock should not be treated with vasopressors, steroids or sodium bicarbonate.

8. It is recommended to use a high-flow fluid warmer to heat crystalloid fluids to 39°C to avoid hypothermia.

9. Electrocardiographic monitoring should be established. If the patient's rhythm is electromechanical dissociation, think cardiac tamponade, tension pneumothorax or profound hypovolaemia.

10. **Disability**: neurologic status – **AVPU** method classifies patients into **a**lert, responds to **v**ocal stimuli, responds only to **p**ainful stimuli or **u**nresponsive. The more extensive Glasgow Coma Scale may be done in the primary or secondary survey. Exclude head injury, decreased oxygenation, shock and altered level of consciousness secondary to alcohol and/or drugs.

11. **Exposure**/environmental control: the patient should be completely undressed by cutting away the garments. Cover the patient in warm blankets and warm intravenous fluids to prevent hypothermia.

12. **Urinary and gastric catheters**: placement of urinary and gastric catheters is considered as part of resuscitation. Urinary catheterization is contraindicated in patients in whom urethral transection is suspected. Suggestive findings include blood at the penile meatus, blood in the scrotum or a prostate gland that is high riding or not palpable. A gastric catheter or nasogastric tube is inserted to reduce gastric distension and decrease the risk of aspiration. If the cribiform plate is fractured or the patient has extensive mid-facial injuries, insert the gastric tube orally to prevent intracranial passage of the tube.

13. **Monitoring**: should include monitoring of the ventilatory rate, arterial blood gases, pulse oximetry, blood pressure and continuous ECG monitoring.

14. **Note**: life-saving measures are initiated when the problem is identified rather than after the primary survey.

15. **X-rays:** in this patient with blunt trauma, a cervical spine, chest (AP) and AP pelvis portable X-ray should be obtained during the primary survey. During the secondary survey, open-mouth odontoid and anteroposterior thoracolumbar films may be obtained with a portable X-ray.

Station 88: Answers

1. Introduce yourself to the patient. Shake her hand. Assess for sweaty palms, which may suggest hyperthyroidism. Establish a rapport.

2. Ask permission to examine her.

3. Ask her if the mass is painful.

4. Inspect the patient's general appearance. Does she have coarse hair, exophthalmos, peaches and cream complexion or pre-tibial myxoedema? Is she thin or obese?

5. Look at the neck. Are there any scars? Is there a tracheal stoma? Is the mass obviously a goitre?

6. Ask the patient to swallow. Observe the movement of the goitre.

7. Ask the patient to count to ten to assess for stridor, which may indicate tracheal compression.

8. Palpate the trachea. Is it midline?

9. Inform the patient that you are about to examine her neck from behind. Palpate the thyroid gland. Is it soft or firm? Is it diffusely enlarged or nodular? Offer her a glass of water and ask her to sip and hold the water in her mouth. Palpate the thyroid gland from behind and ask her to swallow. Feel the thyroid mass move.

10. Palpate the neck from behind for lymphadenopathy. Start at the mastoid bone and palpate along the line of the trapezius muscle and in the posterior triangle down to the clavicle. Palpate along the anterior line of the sternocleidomastoid muscle down to the suprasternal notch feeling for deep cervical nodes. Palpate up the anterior triangle, feeling the trachea, thyroid gland, laryngeal cartilages and hyoid bone. Assess for trotter's sign (loss of laryngeal crepitus may be a sign of post-cricoid neoplasm). Palpate for the submental, submandibular, parotid, pre-auricular and occipital lymph nodes. If the lymph nodes are palpable, assess whether the nodes are separate (reactive, glandular fever, lymphoma, etc.) or matted (tubercu-

losis, neoplasm), mobile or fixed to the skin, fleshy and rubbery (Hodgkin's disease) or hard (cancerous).

11. If the patient has an obvious goitre, percuss the manubrium. Is it dull to percussion suggesting retrosternal involvement?

12. Auscultate over the thyroid for a bruit.

13. Assuming the patient has an obvious goitre, assess her thyroid status. Check the pulse. Examine the hands. Does she have a tremor? Examine her eyes. Does she have a lid lag? Check her deep tendon reflexes.

14. At the 30-second bell, suggest a likely diagnosis of a multi-nodular goitre with no retrosternal extension, no bruit, no palpable lymph nodes and state that the patient is clinically euthyroid.

15. Thank the patient for her cooperation.

Station 89: Answers

1. Introduce yourself to the patient and establish a rapport.

2. Ask the patient for his permission to examine him.

3. Ask him to lie on the bed (reclined at 45°) with his chest bare.

4. Note the patient's general appearance. Is he obese or emaciated? Is he breathless at rest? Does he use his accessory muscles of respiration? Does he have central cyanosis? Is his breathing noisy? Do you hear wheezy expirations?

5. Ask to see his hands. Does he have clubbing, peripheral cyanosis or nicotine staining of the fingers? Does he have wasting of the intrinsic muscles of the hand. If the patient is cyanosed, check for flapping tremor of the hands or asterixis (CO_2 retention). Feel his pulse.

6. Check for raised venous pressure (cor pulmonale) or distension of the neck veins (superior vena cava obstruction).

7. Examine the trachea in the sternal notch for any deviation or a tracheal tug (descent of trachea with inspiration).

8. Palpate for lymphadenopathy in the cervical and axillary regions.

9. Feel for the apex beat.

10. Assess chest expansion with a tape measure or by placing both hands over the sides of the patient's rib cage. Assess the distance between each thumb and the midline to exclude asymmetry and the distance (in cm) between both thumbs to assess expansion. Normal chest expansion is 5 cm.

11. Percuss the chest and over the axillae.

12. Assess tactile vocal fremitus by applying the ulnar aspect of the hand to the patient's chest and asking the patient to repeat '99'.

13. Auscultate for breath sounds with the bell and then the diaphragm. Ask the patient to open his mouth and breathe in and out slowly and deeply.

14. Check for vocal resonance by asking the patient to repeat '99' and auscultating the chest. Normally, the numbers are muffled

on auscultation and clearer over a consolidated lung. Check for whispering pectoriloquy or whispering speech.

15. Note your findings using the following accepted abbreviations:

Do not forget to write the date and time of examination in the beginning, and both sign and print your name at the end. Use legible handwriting.

RS: JVP ⟷

Trachea ⊥

		Front	Back
Chest	Inspection	NAD	NAD
	Expansion	R = L = normal	R = L = normal
	PN	R = L = RES	R = L = RES
	Auscultation	R L	L R

BS vesicular + NIL

Note that the recognized annotations for other physical findings are as follows:

O/E: General: °JACCOL

CVS: PR: 80 bpm reg, regular rhythm, volume normal, character normal
BP: 120/80
JVP: ⟷
HS: I + II + NIL

RS: (as above)

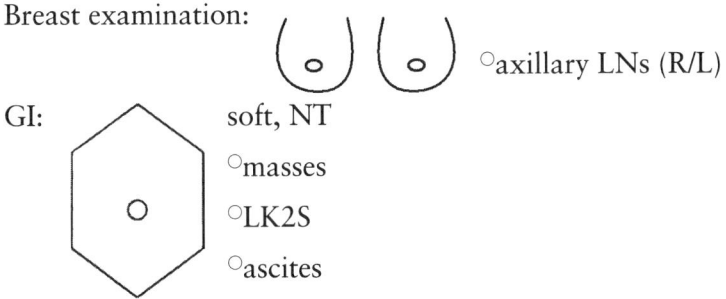

Breast examination: (o) (o) °axillary LNs (R/L)

GI: soft, NT
°masses
°LK2S
°ascites

Auscultation: bowel sounds – normal

NS: (see Station 86)

Station 90: Answers

1. The obvious abnormalities on the blood test are mild hypernatraemia, profound hypokalaemia and mildly elevated levels of bicarbonate (suggestive of metabolic alkalosis). Hypokalaemia is also demonstrated on the ECG by the presence of flattened T-waves.

2. The presence of hypertension, hypokalaemia, alkalosis and a mildly elevated sodium suggest a likely diagnosis of primary hyperaldosteronism. The most common cause of primary hyperaldosteronism is Conn's syndrome, which is caused by an aldosterone secreting adenoma of the adrenal cortex. Symptoms include myasthaenia, polydipsia and polyuria.

3. The next step is to check AM plasma levels of aldosterone, renin and angiotensin. In primary hyperaldosteronism, the aldosterone level is high and the renin level low. In secondary hyperaldosteronism (accelerated hypertension, heart failure, renal artery stenosis, diuretics, etc.), the renin level will also be high.

4. A computed tomographic (CT) scan of the adrenal glands may demonstrate an adrenal adenoma, carcinoma or bilateral adrenal hyperplasia.

5. Treatment for Conn's syndrome involves preoperative spironolactone for 4 weeks before surgery.

Station 91: Answers

1. The obvious abnormalities on the blood tests are anaemia, thrombocytopaenia and the presence of a few immature blast cells on blood film.

2. The most likely diagnosis is acute leukaemia. In this patient, acute myeloid leukaemia, rather than acute lymphoblastic leukaemia, is suggested by the presence of gum hypertrophy.

3. The diagnosis is confirmed by bone marrow examination for a proliferation of blast cells derived from the myeloid elements.

4. Treatment is threefold and involves supportive care with blood and platelet transfusions, chemotherapy with daunorubicin, cytosine arabinoside, and thioguanine and allogeneic bone marrow transplant infused intravenously.

Station 92: Answers

1. Refer to the answer to Station 36 to review the fundamentals of performing a fundoscopic examination.

2. In this scenario, upon looking at the fundus, a slide of papilloedema may be projected.

3. 'This patient has papilloedema as evidenced by. ... The optic disc is swollen forwards and outwards into the surrounding retina. The disc margins are blurred. The retinal veins are congested and there are a few haemorrhages.'

4. The most likely cause for the patient's papilloedema is raised intracranial pressure from head trauma.

5. Other causes of papilloedema include raised intracranial pressure (meningoencephalitis, haemorrhage-subdural, extradural, subarachnoid, intracranial, cerebral oedema), malignant hypertension, optic neuritis, central retinal vein thrombosis, benign intracranial hypertension and metabolic causes.

Station 93: Answers

1. Introduce yourself to the patient and establish a rapport.

2. The aim is to reassure, inform and obtain written consent from the patient.

3. The GMC's guidelines are detailed in the booklet *Seeking Patient's Consent: The Ethical Considerations*. The guidelines are as given below.

4. **Providing sufficient information**: patients have a right to information about their condition and the treatment options available to them.

5. **Details of the diagnosis and prognosis, and the likely prognosis if the condition is left untreated.** Explain to the patient that he has a hernia that needs repair (his diagnosis), and that the likely prognosis if the hernia is left untreated is the risk that it may become irreducible or strangulate and cause bowel obstruction, ischaemia and ultimately become gangrene.

6. **Explain any uncertainties about the diagnosis including options for further investigation before treatment.** In this case, explain that the diagnosis was made on history and clinical examination.

7. **Offer options for treatment or management of the condition, including the option not to treat.** In this situation, explain that the treatment options are conservative (do nothing or wear a truss) and surgical.

8. **Explain the purpose of the treatment; details of the procedure involved, including subsidiary treatment such as methods of pain relief; how the patient should prepare for the procedure; and details of what the patient might experience after the procedure including common and serious side-effects.** Offer details of the operation. For instance, explain that he is having a Lichtenstein mesh repair of the hernia. This operation involves making a small surgical incision in his right groin, opening and reducing the hernia sac, and securing a piece of prosthetic mesh in the groin to prevent recurrence of the hernia. Explain that he must not eat or drink after midnight the day before the operation but that it is important that he take his morning medication with a sip of water.

9. **Offer explanations of the likely benefits and the probability of success; and discussion of any serious or frequently occurring risks, and of any lifestyle changes which may be caused or necessitated by the treatment.** The advantage of this method of hernia repair is that it can be performed under local anaesthesia in the Day Surgery Unit. This is advisable in his case, as his multiple medical conditions put him at higher risk if the operation were to be performed under a general anaesthetic. Explain that this technique carries a low risk of failure. The complications of this operation include infection, haematoma, urinary retention, exacerbation of prostatic symptoms and recurrence. Reassure the patient that the Lichtenstein mesh technique is associated with fewer complications than other techniques of hernia repair.

10. Explain that as the operation will be performed under a local rather than general anaesthesia, he is at lower risk for developing urinary retention and a deep venous thrombosis. He will also have less cardiac or circulatory risks inherent in a general anaesthetic.

11. Explain that as the operation is a day case, that he will need to arrange for someone to pick him up and drive him home on the evening of the operation. Explain that he will be sent home with analgesia and that any external stitches will need to be removed in 5–7 days by the nurse practitioner at his local general practice.

12. **Inform the patient of the name of the doctor who will have overall responsibility for the treatment and, where appropriate, the names of the senior members of his or her team.**

13. **Inform the patient whether doctors in training will be involved.**

14. **Remind the patient that he can change his mind about his decision at any time and that he has a right to seek a second opinion.**

15. Ask the patient if he has any questions.

16. Offer him the completed written consent form to read. If he is agreeable, explain that he should print his name, sign and date the form where indicated.

Station 94: Answers

1. Introduce yourself to Mrs Kahn and establish a rapport.

2. The aim of this discussion is to find out what the husband wants and enable him to do it, and to harmonize with the family's wishes. Also, find out what the husband's and family's hopes and fears are.

3. Explain that the options for terminal care include care in a hospital setting, care at a hospice or care at home. Ask Mrs Khan what she and her husband would like. She confirms that they are in agreement that he should be cared for at home.

4. Ask her what her husband's and family's hopes and fears are. Attempt to reassure her.

5. Explain that it will be important to determine each pain that her husband may experience so that appropriate medication can be prescribed for him at home. For instance, bone pain is treated with opiates such as diamorphine. The diamorphine is titrated to the level of pain and once the required dose is known, a twice-daily dose of a slow-releasing morphine drug (MST) can be administered. Laxatives and antiemetics are prescribed to alleviate the potential side-effects of opioids. Anti-inflammatory drugs such as naproxen are also useful to alleviate bone pain.

6. Empathize with her bereavement. Explain that the normal grieving process includes numbness → denial → yearning → depression → guilt and aggression → reintegration or acceptance. Explain that this process may take years and may require counselling for her and her family.

7. Explain that the family will not be alone at home and that available assistance include her GP, the community and hospice nurses, friends and neighbours, night nurses, vicar, health visitor, and CRUSE (help for the widowed).

8. Ask her if she has any questions. Inform her that she, her husband and her family should feel free to contact you at the hospital if future questions or issues arise.

Station 95: Answers

1. Refer to the answer to Station 36 to review the fundamentals of fundoscopic examination.

2. 'The obvious abnormalities on inspection of the patient's fundi are the presence of blot haemorrhages, micro-aneuryms, tortuous and congested veins, and hard exudates (lipid deposition on the retina). This patient has background diabetic retinopathy.'

3. When examining the diabetic eye, be wary of signs of abducens palsy, cataracts and rubeosis (new vessel formation on the iris).

4. The other type of diabetic retinopathy is proliferative retinopathy. The changes consistent with this condition include:
   - any of the above found in background retinopathy;
   - neovascularization (new vessel formation over the optic disc and the nerves);
   - soft exudates (cotton wool spots that result from infarction of the inner layers of the retina); and
   - flame-shaped haemorrhages (ischaemic changes) and circinate rings of hard exudates (oedema).

   Treatment for proliferative retinopathy is photocoagulation.

5. In advanced diabetic eye disease, vitreous (subhyaloid) haemorrhages, scarring and retinal detachment may also be present. Diabetic retinopathy is a common cause of blindness in the adult population.

Station 96: Answers

1. Introduce yourself to the patient and establish a rapport.

2. Start with an open-ended question. Ask her to explain to you what the problem is and how you can help her.

3. Maintain good eye contact.

4. Notice non-verbal and verbal cues. Be sympathetic.

5. Establish whether she is experiencing the symptoms associated with anxiety neurosis. Has she suffered from symptoms of hyperventilation, headache, sweating, palpitations, tingling in her fingers, poor appetite, a lump in the throat when she swallows saliva (globus hystericus), difficulty in falling asleep, etc.

6. Ask about any repetitive thoughts (obsessions) or compulsive activities.

7. Determine the type of anxiety the patient is experiencing. Is she in a continuous state of anxiety that fluctuates in response to environmental circumstances? Or does she experience sudden panic attacks with physical symptoms? Or does she suffer from phobic anxiety? Or does she have an anxious personality?

8. Have the patient over breathe for 2–3 minutes to recreate the symptoms of a panic attack. Does rebreathing in a paper bag alleviate the symptoms? When does she have these panic attacks? Is she at risk for hypoglycaemia? Does she skip breakfast or exercise excessively?

9. Determine the cause of her anxiety. Ask her about her family and home atmosphere. Is there stress at home? Is anyone at home ill? Is there marital discord?

10. Have there been any significant life events? Is she working? Has she moved house or changed jobs? Has someone close recently passed away?

11. Ask about any medication she has been taking. Is she taking sleeping tablets or diazepam? Withdrawal of benzodiazepines may result in acute anxiety or psychotic symptoms arising 1–2

weeks later. Symptoms may include insomnia, hyperactivity, panic attacks, irritability and depression.

12. Ask her about her social habits. Exclude alcohol and drug dependence. Does she smoke or drink alcohol and, if so, how much? Does she drink tea or coffee and, if so, how many cups a day?

13. Ask about her previous psychiatric history. Does she have a history of depression?

14. Ask about any family history of schizophrenia.

15. Ask about her medical history. Does she suffer from hyperthyroidism or pheochromocytoma (two causes of anxiety neurosis)?

16. Do not rush in and prescribe benzodiazepines. Suggest avoiding caffeinated beverages in the evening and offer relaxation exercises for bedtime.

17. Offer her psychotherapy, progressive relaxation training, and/or hypnosis.

Station 97: Answers

1. Introduce yourself to the patient and establish a rapport.

2. Explain that based on the history and clinical findings, you would like to establish whether she has a healthy intrauterine pregnancy or whether the pregnancy has taken place in her right Fallopian tube instead. This would be an ectopic or extrauterine pregnancy meaning a pregnancy that has occurred outside the womb.

3. Explain to her that you would like to take blood for full blood count, type and cross (to determine her blood group and Rhesus status), and serum β-HCG and progesterone levels. The latter will aid you in determining whether the pregnancy is viable or not.

4. Explain that you would like to take a high vaginal swab to exclude infection as she has a bloody vaginal discharge.

5. Explain that you would like to arrange an urgent transvaginal ultrasound that day to determine whether the pregnancy has occurred in the womb or elsewhere. The scan will also assess the right iliac fossa for appendicitis or ovarian pathology, if a viable intrauterine pregnancy is demonstrated. Avoid medical jargon when addressing the patient.

6. Explain that if the scan reveals a live ectopic pregnancy, she will need to be admitted for emergency laparoscopy and proceed to remove the ectopic from her Fallopian tube. This is a life-threatening condition. If left untreated, the foetus will enlarge and rupture her Fallopian tube, causing massive internal haemorrhage.

7. Explain that if the scan shows no intrauterine pregnancy and the HCG level comes back as < 1500, she will need to have a repeat HCG and progesterone in 48 hours. If the HCG level does not double, it is more than likely that she has an ectopic that is too small to detect at this stage or a non-viable pregnancy.

8. Explain to her that having an ectopic pregnancy puts her at 10% risk of having another ectopic and does diminish her

chances of having a healthy intrauterine pregnancy due to tubal damage. The rates quoted suggest that only one-third of women proceed to have an intrauterine pregnancy.

9. Ask the patient if she has any questions.

Station 98: Answers

1. Introduce yourself to the patient and establish a rapport.

2. Explain that you have received the results of his pre-operative blood tests. Explain that the blood tests suggest that alcohol intake is affecting his blood cells and liver function.

3. Remember the mnemonic 'CONTROL' as you probe into the extent of his alcohol intake:

- 'Can you always control your drinking?'

- 'Has alcohol ever led you to neglect your family or your work?'

- 'What time do you start drinking?'

- 'Do friends comment on how much you drink or ask you to reduce your intake?'

- 'Do you ever drink in the mornings to overcome a hangover?'

- 'Go through an average day's alcohol, leaving nothing out.' More than 3 units day^{-1}.

- Acceptable alcohol intake for a woman is < 15 units week^{-1} and for a man < 20 units week^{-1}. One unit is the equivalent of a glass of wine or half a pint of beer.

4. Ask the patient if he has ever been convicted of assault, driving offences or child neglect. Has he ever attempted suicide or suffered depression?

5. Explain that alcohol has an adverse effect on all organs of the body. It causes hepatitis and cirrhosis in the liver, cortical atrophy, seizures, psychosis, and encephalopathy in the brain, arrhythmias and cardiomyopathy in the heart, peptic ulcers and pancreatitis in the gut, etc.

6. Suggest tips to cut-down alcohol consumption. Consume more non-alcoholic beverages or alcohol-free beer. Limit drinking to social occasions. Do not buy yourself a drink when it is your turn to buy a round of drinks. Go out to the pub later. Take 'rest days' from alcohol. Learn to say 'no'. Suggest keeping an alcohol diary. Suggest that he involve his family.

7. Offer information on group therapy, self-help groups such as Alcoholics Anonymous, treatment units, local and community alcohol teams, and disulfiram (antabuse) treatment.

8. Ask the patient if he has any questions or would like any points clarified.

Station 99: Answers

1. Introduce yourself to the patient and her mother and establish a rapport.

2. Explain that as trimethoprim and benzamycin gel has not been tolerated, that you would like to suggest alternate treatment with minocin MR (minocycline), dianette and differin gel for 3 months.

3. Explain that minocin MR is a once a day antibiotic in the tetracycline class. Explain that the advantage of this antibiotic is that it offers less likelihood of bacterial resistance. Bacterial resistance is associated with other antibiotics used for acne treatment such as erythromycin. Explain that as the patient has all her adult teeth present, she is not at risk for tooth discoloration that has been associated with tetracycline use. Explain that the reported side-effects of minocin MR occur with > 6 months use and include liver damage and systemic lupus erythematosis. She will only be taking the antibiotic for 3 months and so should not be at risk. Other reported side-effects include dizziness, rash or pigmentation. If this should occur, the drug should be discontinued.

4. Explain that the second pill is called dianette. Explain that it is both a form of hormonal therapy for acne and a combined oral contraceptive. Explain that the advantage is that it is licensed to be used for the treatment of acne in cases that have shown resistance to antibiotics. Contraindications to the use of this drug include a history of migraines with a focal aura, hypertension, smoking, a family history of arterial disease or venous thromboembolism in a first-degree relative aged < 45. The reported side-effects include nausea, vomiting, headaches, breast tenderness, fluid retention and reduced menstrual flow. This does not imply that she will necessarily experience any or all of these side-effects. If she does experience any of these side-effects, she should consult her GP. The patient is to take one tablet a day from day 1 of her menstrual cycle for 21 days and then have a 7-day pill-free period before starting a new pack.

5. Explain that the differin (adapalene) gel is a topical retinoid and is used to treat mild to moderate acne. It is to be applied in a thin layer to the areas of acne at bedtime. Reported side-effects include local reactions such as stinging, burning, erythema or peeling skin. If this occurs, the drug should be

discontinued. The patient's skin will be sensitive to UVB light and sunlight.

6. Ask the patient and mother if they have any questions or whether they need anything clarified.

7. Hand them the prescription.

8. Ask them to make a follow-up appointment for 3 months time.

Station 100: Answers

1. Introduce yourself to the patient and establish a rapport.

2. Discuss the presenting complaint. Is the right-sided loin pain and haematuria acute or recurrent? Ask her to describe the pain. How severe is the pain? Is it a dull ache or sharp in nature? Does it radiate? Does anything alleviate or aggravate the pain? Has she taken any painkillers?

3. Ask questions aimed at narrowing the potential list of differential diagnoses for macroscopic haematuria. Consider all renal, extrarenal and systemic causes. Has she suffered from kidney stones in the past? Does she have a history of urinary tract infections? Has she been involved in an accident or received injury (blunt trauma) to her kidneys or bladder?

4. Does she or anyone in her family have a history of bleeding dyscrasias or coagulopathies?

5. Is she on a blood-thinning drug such as warfarin or aspirin?

6. The most likely diagnosis for this patient with hypertension, renal impairment, large and irregular kidneys, acute loin pain, and macroscopic haematuria is adult polycystic renal disease. This is an autosomal-dominant condition and, therefore, counselling is suggested for relatives of affected individuals. An abdominal X-ray may exclude the presence of radio-opaque renal calculi. Definitive diagnosis is made on ultrasound scan of the kidneys.